INTRODUCTION TO ELECTROCARDIOGRAPHY

INTRODUCTION TO ELECTROCARDIOGRAPHY

PAUL L. HUANG, MD, PhD
Instructor, Harvard Medical School
Cardiac Unit, Medical Services
Massachusetts General Hospital
Boston, Massachusetts

W.B. SAUNDERS COMPANY
Harcourt Brace Jovanovich, Inc.

Philadelphia London Toronto Montreal Sydney Tokyo

W. B. SAUNDERS COMPANY
Harcourt Brace Jovanovich, Inc.

The Curtis Center
Independence Square West
Philadelphia, Pennsylvania 19106

Library of Congress Cataloging-in-Publication Data

Huang, Paul L.
　　Introduction to electrocardiography / Paul L. Huang.
　　　　p.　　cm.
　　ISBN 0-7216-4856-8
　　1. Electrocardiography.　　I. Title.
　　[DNLM: 1. Electrocardiography.　　WG 140 H872i]
　RC683.5.E5H75　　1993
　616.1′2—dc20
　DNLM/DLC
　　　　　　　　　　　　　　　　　　　　　　　　　　　　　　92-49603

Introduction to Electrocardiography　　　　　　　　　ISBN 0-7216-4856-8

Copyright © 1993 by W. B. Saunders Company.

All rights reserved. No part of this publication may be reproduced or transmitted in any form or by any means, electronic or mechanical, including photocopy, recording, or any information storage and retrieval system, without permission in writing from the publisher.

Printed in the United States of America.

Last digit is the print number:　　9　　8　　7　　6　　5　　4　　3　　2　　1

FOREWORD

In 1903, Einthoven, using a simple wind-up galvanometer, was the first to record the electrical phenomena of the heart. His pioneering work in electrocardiography brought him the recognition of the Nobel Prize in 1924. Frank N. Wilson, who would later contribute so much to the development of vectorcardiography, wrote in 1952 that "when the press or the radio announces the sudden death of a celebrity from heart disease, a multitude of middle-aged persons runs out to make an electrocardiogram the next morning." The initial importance of cardiac electrical activity in the diagnostic process has evolved over the last three decades into a technological explosion that not only has led to the exact diagnostic and prognostic evaluation of cardiac electrical activity by sophisticated electrophysiological methods but has also brought effective pharmacologic, electrical and surgical treatments for the most serious arrhythmias. Nevertheless, despite such technologic explosion in regard to the diagnostic, prognostic, and management of distorted cardiac electrical activity, it is important to recognize that the appropriate reading of a plain electrocardiogram as developed early in this century is crucial for the appropriate approach to the patient before more sophisticated technology is applied.

When Dr. Paul Huang asked me to write the foreword of his book, *Introduction to Electrocardiography,* on the one hand I felt proud that he chose me since he is one of the most valuable members of our Cardiac Unit, which I was recently asked to direct as the new Chief of Cardiology. On the other hand, before I accepted the task, I wanted to know in depth the content of the book, as is my norm, and for this reason I asked for two weeks to be able to read it in detail. I finished yesterday and today I can write this foreword with great satisfaction.

The first question in regard to a new book on electrocardiography is, is it really necessary? I believe that there are three steps in learning electrocardiography. The first involves a simple method of understanding of the genesis of the different electrocardiographic patterns as they apply to common diseases. The second is a more extensive and detailed approach to electrocardiography and vectorcardiography as it is available in a number of textbooks dedicated to the subject. The third is to be able in daily practice to systematically read an electrocardiogram without making a common mistake—lack of method.

Within this context there are three aspects of Dr. Paul Huang's book that are especially important and support the justification of this new book: (1) It can be used by medical students as a first approach to the understanding of the different electrocardiographic patterns as they apply to the various cardiac disease entities; the student, however, should not expect a lengthy explanation of the mechanisms that lead to the different tracings since this is not the scope of the book. (2) This is an excellent summary for those individuals who are already trained in reading electrocardiography but who want to master a methodologic approach for appropriate and rapid evaluation of tracings, and (3) This is a very clearly written book, the tracings are of excellent quality, and, as stated, it offers a clear approach, with a well-thought-out method.

We should congratulate Dr. Paul Huang for putting together this very concise book that outlines an easy-to-follow systematic approach to electrocardiography that can be of help not only to medical students but also to physicians in their daily practice.

VALENTIN FUSTER, M.D., Ph.D.

PREFACE

Electrocardiography is one of the oldest diagnostic tools used in cardiology. Since it was developed in 1906 by Einthoven, the standard 12-lead electrocardiogram has become an important, rapid, noninvasive technique that yields a surprising amount of information. Despite the abundance of new diagnostic procedures and techniques, the electrocardiogram has, along with the history and physical examination, remained the mainstay of initial cardiac evaluation of the patient.

It is easy to be struck by the most obvious changes present on an ECG, for example, ST-segment elevations that indicate an acute myocardial infarction. However, unless one interprets the tracings carefully and systematically, the shift of the axis to the left, or the second-degree heart block, may not be so immediately apparent. Thus it is helpful to develop a systematic approach to reading ECGs that is always followed.

This book attempts to present a systematic approach to ECG interpretation. For each tracing, this includes the following steps:

Determine the rhythm
Determine the rate
Determine the intervals
Determine the QRS axis
Examine the P waves
Examine the QRS complex
Examine the ST segments
Examine the T waves
Look for evidence of ischemia or infarction

Each chapter covers a specific topic and builds on the previous ones. After completing a chapter, the reader may turn to the ECG tracings in the cases in Section II, and use them to practice the specific topics covered in that lesson. For example, Chapter 2 covers determination of the QRS axis and R-wave progression. After reviewing the material, the reader may go through the ECG tracings, and determine the QRS axis and evaluate the R-wave progression for each tracing.

One exception to the stepwise presentation of material is that the interpretation of cardiac rhythms is covered *after* the fundamentals of pattern recognition. Until that section, it will be useful to determine if a rhythm is regular while reading the rate and intervals.

This book was written as a series of lecture notes and handouts for a class given to Harvard Medical School students as part of their core clerkship in medicine at the Massachusetts General Hospital. The material covered has been chosen carefully and has evolved, by necessity, to cover the most important concepts and the practical points necessary for accurate interpretation of ECGs on the wards. Oversimplifications have been made, in the interest of first developing the framework to interpret tracings. After completing this book, interested readers will have the necessary background to turn to more advanced texts to further hone their skills and to study the nuances of electrocardiography.

Paul L. Huang

*This book is dedicated
to my Mother*

CONTENTS

SECTION I SYSTEMATIC APPROACH TO ECGs 1

1 Leads, Rates, and Intervals 3
2 Axis and R-Wave Progression 9
3 Chamber Enlargement and Hypertrophy 15
4 Bundle Branch Blocks and Hemiblocks 21
5 Ischemia and Infarction 29
6 Review of Systematic Approach 35
7 Approach to Arrhythmias and Conduction Blocks 37
8 Supraventricular Arrhythmias 43
9 Ventricular Arrhythmias and Aberrancy 53
10 Drugs and Metabolic Disorders 57

SECTION II PRACTICE ECG TRACINGS 63

Index 185

ACKNOWLEDGMENTS

I wish to thank Dr. John T. Potts and Dr. Mark Fishman for their continued encouragement and support, and for their invaluable guidance. I express deep appreciation to Dr. Valentin Fuster, for his careful reading of the text and for his support, and to Dr. Leslie Fang, Director of the Medicine Core Clerkship at the Massachusetts General Hospital, for providing me with the opportunity to teach electrocardiography to the third-year medical students. I feel extremely fortunate to be able to learn from such cardiologists as Dr. Roman De Sanctis and Dr. Peter Yurchak, and I thank them for reviewing early drafts of this book. I am also indebted to the ECG Laboratory of the Massachusetts General Hospital for assistance in collecting representative tracings. Finally, I am ever so grateful to Mr. Richard Zorab, Senior Medical Editor, and Ms. Lorraine Kilmer, Manager of Editing, Design, and Production, for their patience, support, and encouragement.

SECTION I

Systematic Approach to ECGs

Chapter 1

LEADS, COMPLEXES, RATES, AND INTERVALS

I. INTRODUCTION

This chapter introduces the basic concepts necessary to interpret standard 12-lead electrocardiograms:
   Leads and electrodes
   Determination of the heart rate
   Complexes in the cardiac cycle
   Intervals

After completing this chapter, you will be able to look at any ECG tracing and

1. Determine the heart rate.
2. Read the PR interval, QRS duration, and QT interval and tell if they are normal or abnormal.

II. LEADS AND ELECTRODES

A. Standard Leads

The surface electrocardiogram measures the heart's electrical activity. The most commonly used system employs 12 leads:
   The limb leads I, II, III, aVR, aVL, and aVF
   The chest or precordial leads V1, V2, V3, V4, V5, and V6

Electrocardiograms are generally taken either as a
   strip, with the leads organized in the order listed above, or as a
   sheet, with the leads organized as shown in Figure 1–1.

SECTION I: SYSTEMATIC APPROACH TO ECGs

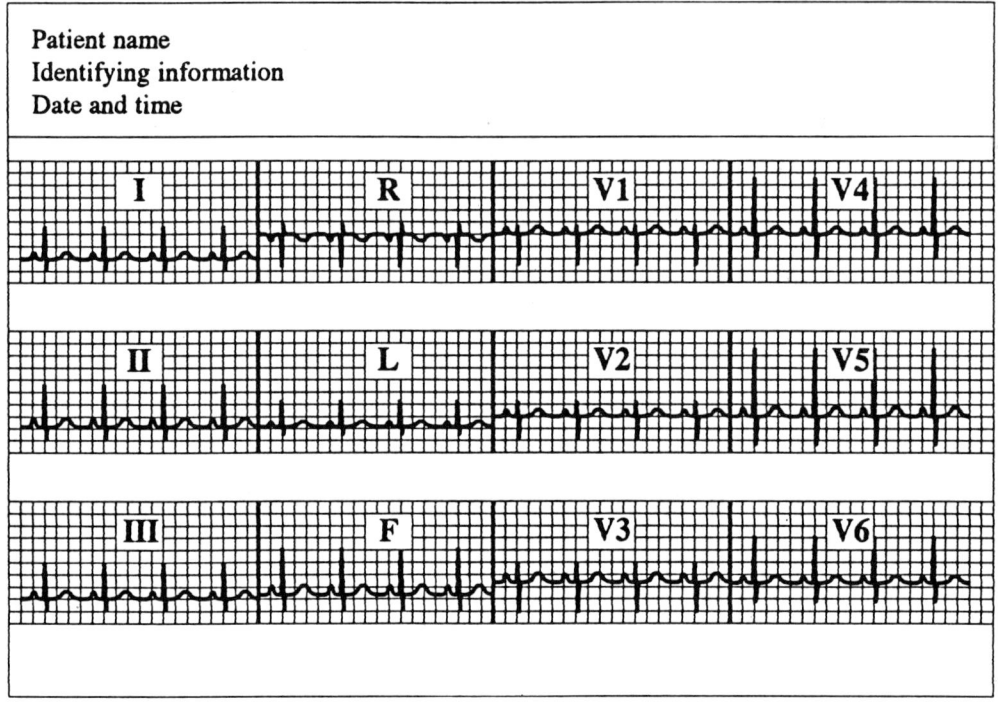

FIGURE 1–1. A 12-lead ECG.

B. Electrodes: How to Take an ECG

In order to take a 12-lead electrocardiogram, you must attach at least five electrodes to the patient's body.

Four color-coded electrodes are attached to the limbs:

Left arm:	black	Right arm:	white
Left leg:	red	Right leg:	green

A useful mnemonic is "*Christmas trees on the feet, green and white on the right.*" From these four limb electrodes, the six limb leads, I, II, III, aVR, aVL, and aVF are derived.

Chest electrodes are placed on the patient's chest in the following positions (see Figure 1–2):

V1: 4th intercostal space, right sternal border
V2: 4th intercostal space, left sternal border
V3: halfway between V2 and V4
V4: 5th intercostal space, midclavicular line
V5: 5th intercostal space, anterior axillary line
V6: 5th intercostal space, midaxillary line

Some machines have six chest electrodes that are individually marked V1 through V6. These machines usually record three leads simultaneously and give tracings as an entire sheet. Other machines have only one chest electrode, which may be placed in each position while that lead is recorded and then moved to the next position. These machines give the tracings in strips.

Even slight differences in lead placement may change the pattern seen on an electrocardiogram. In patients likely to have multiple

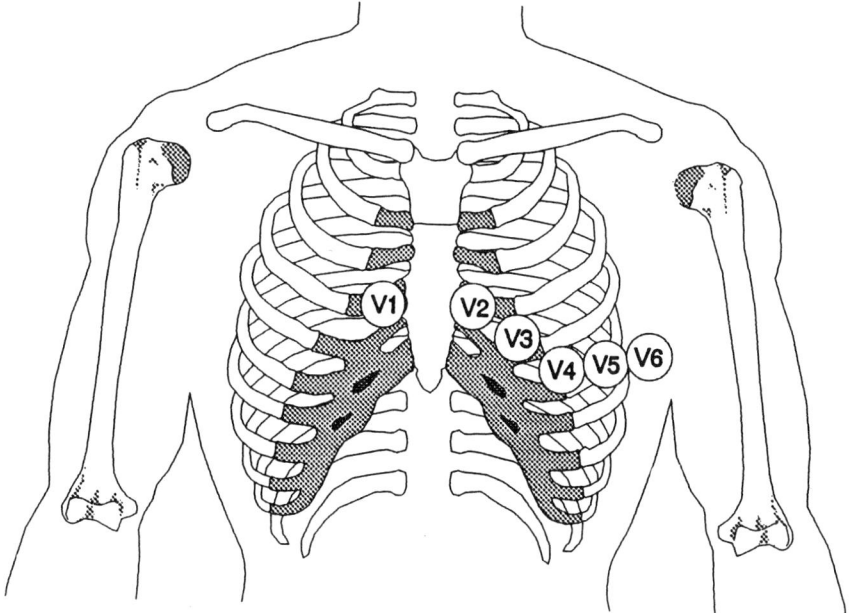

FIGURE 1 2. Placement of chest electrodes.

ECGs and for whom it is important to determine if there are significant changes, for example, in a coronary care unit, it is a good idea to mark the position of the chest electrodes directly on the chest so that differences in lead placement do not complicate interpretation.

The chest electrode also may be used as an exploring electrode. It may be placed over the right side of the chest in a patient with suspected right ventricular infarct or attached to a pericardiocentesis needle to help guide its position.

III. DETERMINATION OF HEART RATE

ECG paper is marked with millimeter grids, and every 5th grid (5 mm) has a boldface dividing line. In this book we will call millimeter grids "small boxes" and the boldface 5-mm divisions "big boxes."

The *vertical axis* of ECGs measures *voltage*. One millimeter (small box) is 1 mV. Each tracing should have a standardization squarewave of 10 mV, which is normally 2 big boxes, or 1 cm, tall. Patients with extremely high voltages may require setting the machine at half-standardization, and those with low voltages may require double-standardization. In these cases, the height of the 10-mV squarewave will tell the standardization.

The *horizontal axis* of ECGs measures *time*. Standard speed for ECG paper is 25 mm/s, so each big box, or 5 mm, represents 0.2s of time. Each small box, or 1 mm, is 0.04s.

To measure intervals, count the number of small boxes in the interval and multiply by 0.04s. For example, if an interval is 3 small boxes, it is 3 × 0.04s, or 0.12s.

6 □ SECTION I: SYSTEMATIC APPROACH TO ECGs

There are two methods for determining the heart rate:

1. For *slow* rates, or *irregular* rates (such as atrial fibrillation), count the number of QRS complexes that occur in 6s, and multiply by 10. On all ECG paper, there are *3-s marks* underneath each strip. The number of QRS complexes that occur in two of these 3-s periods is the number of complexes in 6s.
2. For *regular* rhythms, you can quickly estimate the rate by counting the number of bold boxes that occur between adjacent QRS complexes. It is convenient to start with a complex that lies directly on a bold gridline. The mnemonic is **300–150–100–75–60–50.** You should commit these numbers to memory. For rates that do not fall strictly on the lines, you can interpolate.

Figure 1–3 shows examples of both these methods.

In Figure 1–3A, the rhythm is irregular. There are 7 beats between the two 3-s periods. 7 beats in 6s is 70 beats per minute.

In Figure 1–3B, the rhythm appears regular, so we can use the box-counting method. The third QRS complex falls close to a bold square. Counting to the next QRS complex, we see that the rate is between 75 and 60. We can estimate that the rate is about 70 beats per minute.

Normally, the heart rate is between 60 and 100 beats per minute, although there may be great variability. Rates slower than 60 are defined as bradycardia, and rates greater than 100 are defined as tachycardia.

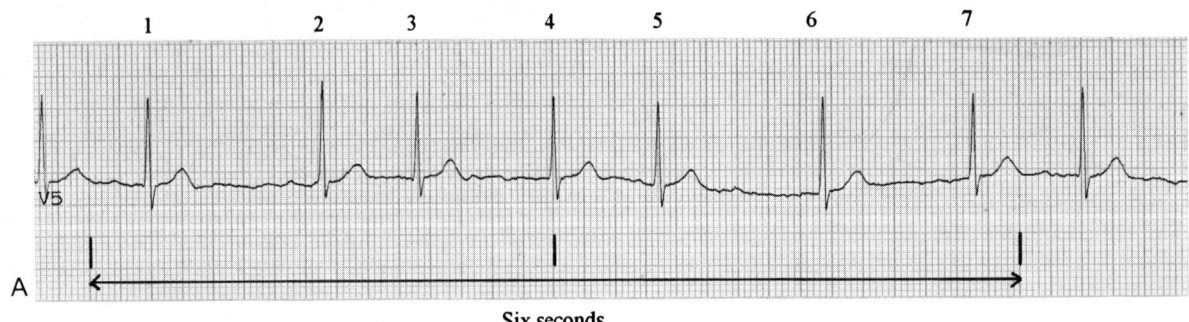
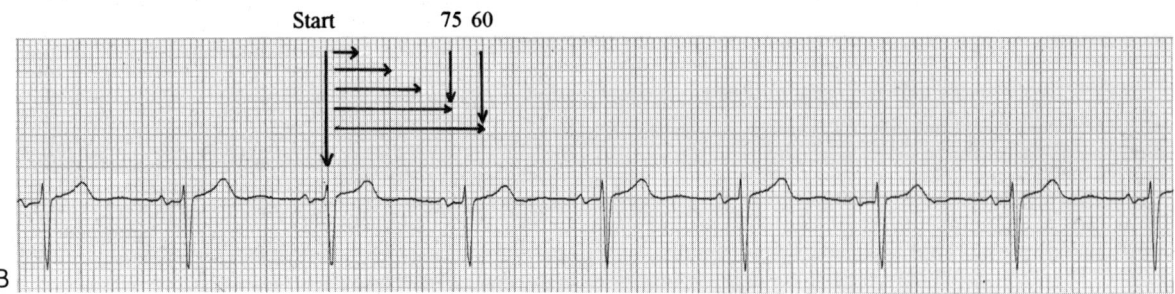

The heart rate is between 75 and 60, about 70

FIGURE 1–3. Determination of heart rate.

IV. COMPLEXES

There are three major complexes in a normal ECG cardiac cycle (see Figure 1–4):
  The *P wave*, corresponding to atrial depolarization
  The *QRS complex*, corresponding to ventricular depolarization
  The *T wave*, corresponding to ventricular repolarization

The atria also repolarize, but the magnitude of this wave is small, and it is usually hidden within the QRS complex.

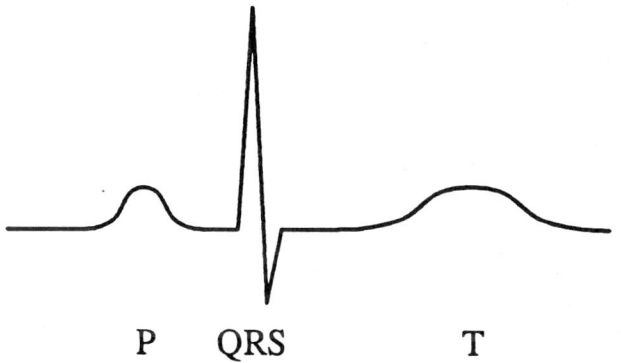

FIGURE 1–4. Complexes in a normal ECG cycle.

A. P Waves

P waves should normally be upright in leads I, II, aVF, and V4–V6. They may give information regarding atrial enlargement. Their absence may suggest atrial fibrillation, junctional rhythm, or ventricular rhythm.

B. QRS Complex

The QRS complex represents depolarization of the left and right ventricles. By definition, the first upward deflection is the R wave. A downward deflection that precedes the R wave is a Q wave. A downward deflection that follows an R wave is an S wave. Not all three components are necessarily present.

The *duration* of the QRS complex is the time it takes for the ventricles to depolarize. A prolonged QRS duration indicates a conduction problem in the ventricles or a bundle-branch block.

The *amplitude* of the QRS complex is also informative. It may be low, suggesting pericardial effusion, myxedema, cardiomyopathy, amyloidosis, or very thick chest wall, or it may be high, suggesting ventricular hypertrophy.

C. T Wave

The T wave represents repolarization of the ventricles. It is normally upright in leads I, II, and V3–V6. It is normally inverted in lead aVR and variable in other leads. Newly inverted T waves may represent ischemia or infarction. Very tall T waves may represent ischemia, acute infarction, or severe hyperkalemia.

V. INTERVALS

Normally, one measures three intervals (see Figure 1–5):
  The *PR interval*
  The *QRS duration*
  The *QT interval*

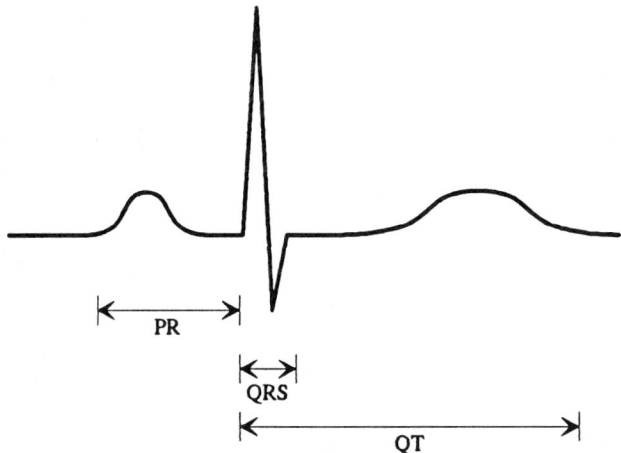

FIGURE 1–5. Intervals in a normal ECG cycle.

The ST segment is important, although the interval itself is not routinely measured.

In measuring intervals, only use the limb leads, and look for the lead where the longest interval is obtained.

A. PR Interval

The PR interval is measured from the *beginning* of the P wave to the *beginning* of the QRS complex. It represents the time it takes for an impulse to travel from the sinus node to the ventricular tissue. Normally, the PR interval is 0.12 to 0.20s (three to five small boxes). Short PR intervals are seen in fast heart rates, in low atrial or junctional rhythms, and where there is a bypass tract, as in Wolf-Parkinson-White syndrome. Long PR intervals are seen in conduction system disease and AV block.

B. QRS Duration

The QRS duration is measured from the *beginning* of the QRS complex to the *end* of the QRS complex. It represents the time it takes for the ventricles to depolarize. The QRS duration is usually 0.04 to 0.10s (one to two and a half small boxes). If it is 0.12s (three boxes) or greater, there is a bundle-branch block. If it is between 0.10s and 0.12s, there is an incomplete bundle-branch block or an interventricular conduction delay.

C. QT Interval

The QT interval is measured from the *beginning* of the QRS complex to the *end* of the T wave. This definition is not intuitively obvious. The QT interval reflects the total duration of ventricular systole—depolarization as well as repolarization. The length of the QT interval is dependent on the rate—the faster the rate, the shorter the normal QT interval. There are tables that list normal QT intervals for different heart rates. A *corrected QT interval*, or *QT_c*, adjusts the QT interval to account for faster or slower heart rates. It is calculated by dividing the measured QT interval by the square root of the R-R interval measured in seconds:

$$QT_c = \frac{QT}{\sqrt{\text{R-R interval}}}$$

At a heart rate of 60 beats per minute, the R-R interval is 1s, and the measured QT interval is the same as the corrected QT interval.

Instead of routinely calculating QT intervals, we will assume that for normal heart rates, a QT interval of 0.28 to 0.40s is normal.

The QT interval is lengthened by many factors, importantly by drugs such as phenothiazines and tricyclic antidepressants, which may predispose to serious ventricular arrhythmias.

VI. SUMMARY

For each tracing, you should be able to do the following:

1. *Determine the rate and whether the rhythm is regular.*
   For most tracings, count the number of large boxes from one QRS complex to another; remember the mnemonic **300–150–100–75–60–50.**
   For irregular rhythms or extremely fast or slow rhythms, count the number of QRS complexes in 6s and multiply by 10.
2. *Calculate the PR interval, QRS duration, and QT interval and decide if they are normal or not.*
   The PR interval should be 0.12 to 0.20s.
   The QRS duration should be less than 0.10s.
   The QT interval should be 0.28 to 0.40s for most heart rates.

Chapter 2

AXIS AND R-WAVE PROGRESSION

I. INTRODUCTION

This chapter describes how to determine the QRS axis and evaluate R-wave progression for any ECG tracing. *QRS axis* refers to the position of the electrical impulse of ventricular depolarization in the frontal plane, determined from the limb leads I, II, III, aVR, aVL, and aVF. *R-wave progression,* on the other hand, refers to how the QRS complex changes from V1 to V6 across the chest leads.

After completing this chapter, you will be able to

1. Decide if the QRS complex is in the normal quadrant or not.
2. Determine the QRS axis numerically and whether it demonstrates left-axis deviation or right-axis deviation.
3. Evaluate R-wave progression and decide if it is normal, poor, or too good.

II. QRS AXIS

A. Determination of Axis

The axis of a QRS complex describes the position of the vector of the electrical impulse in the frontal plane. The position is described as an angle. Normally, ventricular depolarization occurs downward from the atrioventricular (AV) node toward the apex. Thus a normal QRS axis points downward and to the left.

By convention, 0 degrees is defined as horizontal and to the left, and +90 degrees is directly down (see Figure 2–1).

An axis that falls between 0 and +90 degrees is in the normal quadrant. An axis that falls between +90 and +180 degrees is in the rightward axis quadrant, and an axis that falls between 0 and −90 degrees is in the leftward axis quadrant. An axis between −90 degrees and 180 degrees can be considered in the extreme left or extreme right axis quadrant.

The six limb leads are derived from the electrodes placed on the arms and legs. Their relative position is shown in Figure 2–1.

An electrical impulse shows the greatest deflection in leads that are *parallel* to its direction and the smallest deflection in leads that are *perpendicular*. A lead in the exact direction of the axis would have a very positive deflection, whereas a lead directly opposite to the axis would be very negative.

A lead directly perpendicular to the axis would be *isoelectric* and be as positive as it is negative. In general, the QRS also will have the least amplitude in the isoelectric lead.

To determine the axis of a QRS complex, follow these two steps:

Step 1

Determine which quadrant the axis is in. Look at leads I and aVF. By deciding if the complex is positive or negative in these leads, you can tell which quadrant the axis lies in.

Step 2

Look for the isoelectric lead, the lead in which the complex has equal amounts of positive and negative deflections. The QRS axis is 90 degrees to the isoelectric lead. Based on the quadrant the axis is in, decide what the axis is.

As an example, in Case 13 in Section II, the QRS complex in leads I and aVF are both positive, so the QRS axis falls within the normal quadrant. The QRS complex is most isoelectric in lead aVL, which is located at −30 degrees. The axis is 90 degrees to the isoelectric lead aVL and is thus +60 degrees.

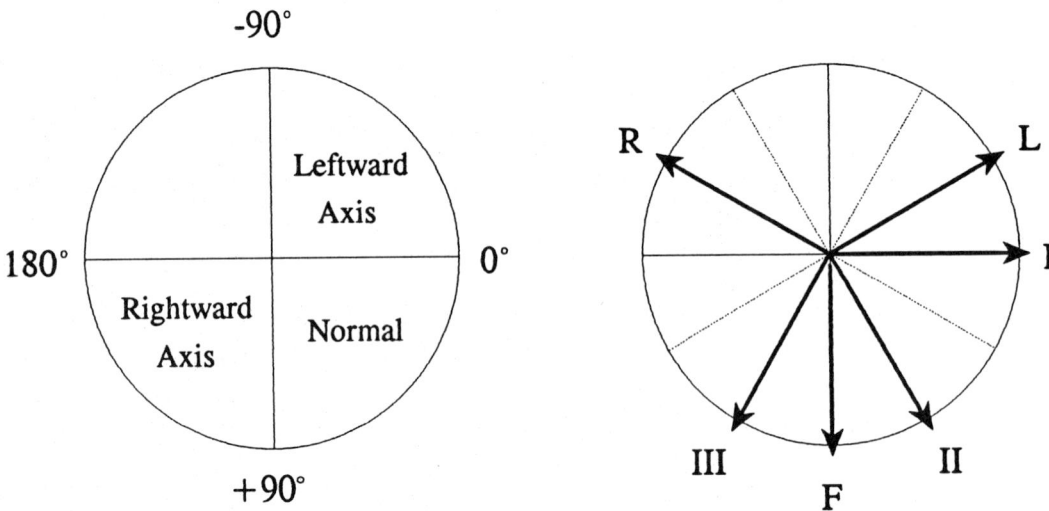

FIGURE 2–1. Definition of quadrants and positions of frontal leads.

In Case 1, the QRS complex is positive in lead I but negative in aVF. This means the axis is in the leftward axis quadrant. The QRS complex is most isoelectric in lead II, which is located at +60 degrees. The axis is 90 degrees to the isoelectric lead II and is thus −30 degrees.

B. Normal and Abnormal QRS Axis

The range of normal QRS axis extends beyond the normal quadrant. QRS axes between −30 and +100 degrees are considered normal (see Figure 2–2).

Left axis deviation (LAD) is defined as an axis in the leftward axis quadrant that is more negative than −30 degrees. An axis between 0 and −30 degrees is simply called *leftward axis,* to distinguish it from left axis deviation, which is considered abnormal.

Right axis deviation (RAD) occurs when the axis is in the rightward axis quadrant and more positive than 100 degrees.

These are some causes of abnormal axis:

Right Axis Deviation

Normal variant
Mechanical shifts: inspiration, emphysema
Right ventricular hypertrophy
Right bundle-branch block
Left posterior hemiblock
Wolff-Parkinson-White syndrome
Dextrocardia
Ventricular ectopy

Left Axis Deviation

Normal variant
Mechanical shifts: expiration, high diaphragm
Left ventricular hypertrophy
Left bundle-branch block
Left anterior hemiblock
Wolff-Parkinson-White syndrome
Endocardial cushion defects
Ventricular ectopy

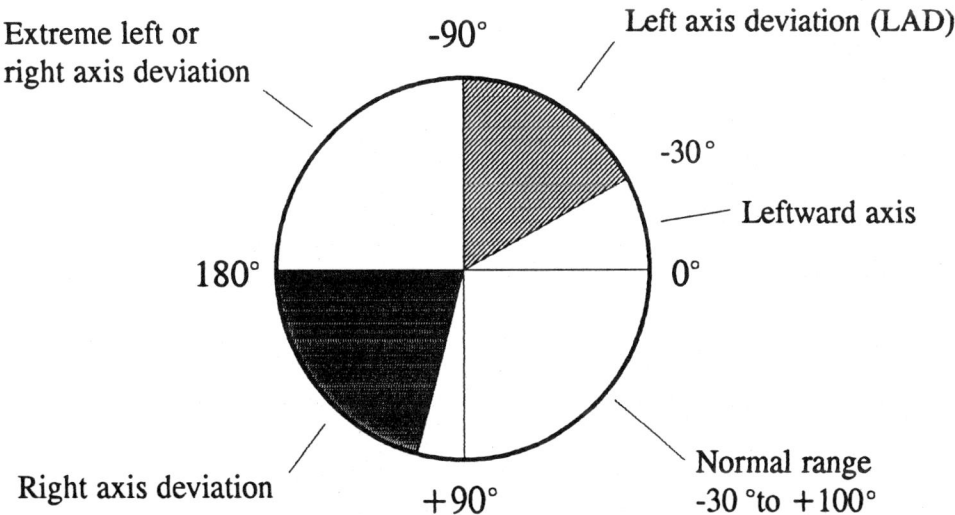

FIGURE 2–2. Normal and abnormal QRS axis.

III. R-WAVE PROGRESSION

While the QRS axis describes the electrical vector in the frontal plane, *R-wave progression* describes the vector across the front of the chest. Strictly speaking, the chest leads do not describe a plane. The phrase *across the precordium* refers to the leads V1 through V6.

Over the normal heart, the R waves get taller as the electrode is moved from right to left across the chest. This occurs because the major sequence of electrical activity is from right to left.

A. Appearance of the QRS Complex in the Chest Leads (Figure 2–3)

The first step of ventricular depolarization is septal depolarization, which occurs normally from left to right. Thus, in lead V1, which overlies the right ventricle, there is an initial small upward deflection. In lead V6, which overlies the left ventricular apex, there is a small downward deflection.

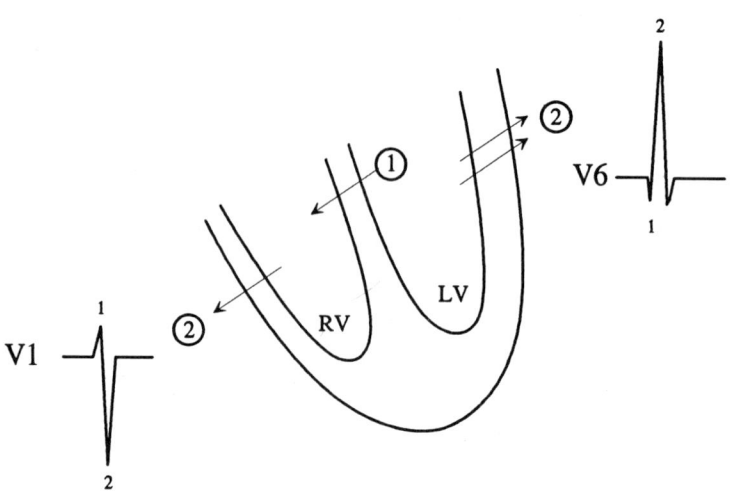

FIGURE 2–3. Appearance of QRS complex in chest leads.

Next, the right and left ventricles depolarize simultaneously. The left ventricle is much thicker than the right, and its contribution to the QRS complex outweighs that of the right ventricle. Thus, in V1, there is a large negative deflection, and in V6, there is a large positive deflection.

The small initial downward deflections noted in lead V6 are called *septal q waves*, because they are the result of septal depolarization. The septum depolarizes away from lead V6, so the deflection is negative. A small *q* is used, to distinguish these normal *q* waves from the pathologic Q waves seen in infarction. Do not confuse *septal q waves*, which are seen in V5 and V6, with changes in the *anteroseptal leads*, V1 and V2.

B. Components of Normal R-Wave Progression

There are two components of *normal* R-wave progression:

1. The R wave of the QRS complex should grow in size from V1 to its peak, between V4 and V6.
2. The *transition zone*, where the QRS goes from predominantly negative to positive, should occur at lead V3 or V4.

If the QRS complex stays negative past V4, there is *poor* R-wave progression.

If the QRS complex is positive before V3, the R-wave progression is said to be *"too good."*

C. Rotation

One of the reasons for abnormal R-wave progression is rotation of the heart relative to the chest. The terms *clockwise rotation* and *counterclockwise rotation* are used to describe rotation of the heart's position in the chest in the horizontal plane.

By convention, one looks up at the heart from below the diaphragm, much like a CT scan image, where one is looking at the cross section toward the patient's head. Rotation to the left would be *clockwise rotation*, and rotation to the right would be *counterclockwise rotation* (Figure 2–4).

Clockwise rotation of a normal heart would give the appearance

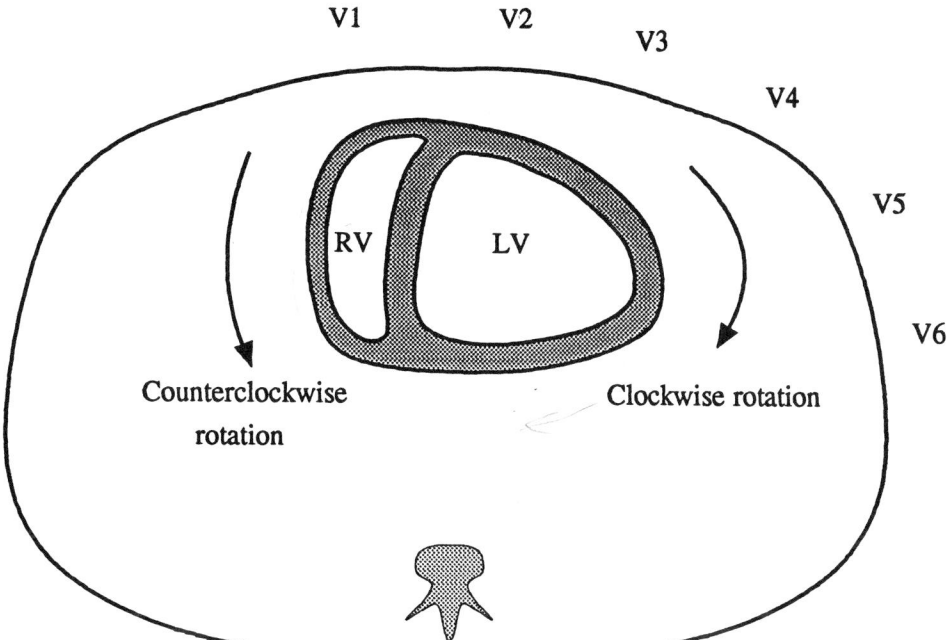

FIGURE 2-4. Rotation of the heart relative to the chest leads.

of poor R-wave progression. Counterclockwise rotation would similarly give the appearance of R-wave progression that is too good, in that the complex may be mostly positive in V1 or V2.

D. Interpretation of R-Wave Progression

The reasons for *poor R-wave progression* include
  Clockwise rotation
  Anteroseptal myocardial infarction (MI)
  Anterior MI
  Left bundle-branch block

The reasons for *tall R waves in leads V1 or V2* (or R-wave progression that is "too good") include
  Counterclockwise rotation
  Right bundle-branch block
  True posterior MI
  Right ventricular hypertrophy
  Wolff-Parkinson-White syndrome.

We will cover these topics in later chapters.

IV. SUMMARY

For each electrocardiogram, you should now be able to

1. Determine the rate.
2. Calculate the PR interval, the QRS duration, and the QT interval.

3. *Determine the quadrant of the QRS axis.* Look to see if the QRS is up or down in leads I and aVF.
4. *Determine the QRS axis in degrees.* Find the isoelectric lead, the lead where the QRS is as positive as it is negative. The axis is 90 degrees to the isoelectric lead.
5. *Look at the R-wave progression and tell if it is normal, poor, or "too good."* Remember the two components of normal R wave progression:

The R wave should grow in size from V1 to its peak at V4 to V6.

The QRS should go from mostly negative to mostly positive at V3 or V4.

Chapter 3

CHAMBER ENLARGEMENT AND HYPERTROPHY

I. INTRODUCTION

This chapter examines the electrocardiographic signs of atrial enlargement and ventricular hypertrophy.

After completing this chapter, you will be able to

1. Look at the P-wave morphology and size in leads II and V1 and decide if there is evidence for left atrial enlargement (LAE) or right atrial enlargement (RAE).
2. Examine the QRS complex for evidence of left ventricular hypertrophy (LVH) and right ventricular hypertrophy (RVH).

II. ATRIAL ENLARGEMENT

Normally, the right atrium (RA) depolarizes momentarily before the left atrium (LA), so the first half of the P wave reflects the RA and the second half reflects the LA.

Atrial depolarization occurs downward, and the normal P-wave axis is +60 degrees, so the P wave is usually most positive in lead II.

Atria generally *enlarge* when they are subjected to volume or pressure overload; they do not *hypertrophy*. The best leads to see the changes of atrial enlargement are II and V1. Let's consider how the normal P wave looks in these leads and then the changes to expect in atrial enlargement.

A. P Waves in Lead II

Normal P-wave morphology in lead II is due to the sum of the depolarization of the RA and the LA. RA depolarization precedes LA depolarization, but the two overlap, to produce a smooth P wave (Figure 3–1A).

In atrial enlargement, two things occur:

1. Depolarization of the enlarged atrium takes longer time.
2. Depolarization of the enlarged atrium results in a slightly bigger contribution to the P wave (more voltage).

In *right atrial enlargement* (*RAE*), the P wave becomes tall and

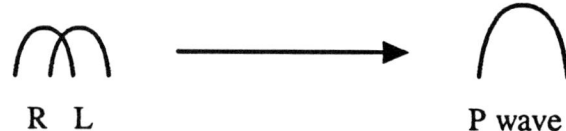

A *Lead II: Normal P wave*

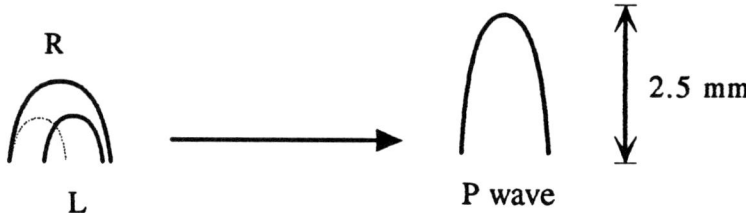

B *Lead II: Right atrial enlargement*

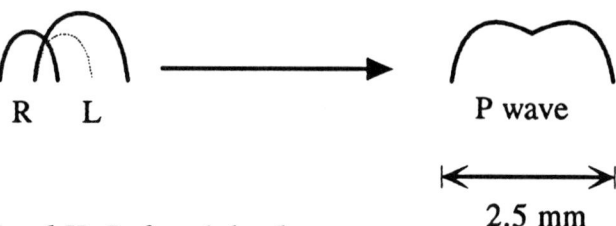

Lead II: Left atrial enlargement

FIGURE 3–1. P wave morphology in lead II.

peaked (Figure 3–1B). The larger voltage of the RA and the longer duration of depolarization results in a taller P wave when overlapped with the contribution from the LA. The duration of the entire P wave (both RA and LA) is not necessarily increased, since they overlap.

*Standard criterion for RAE in lead II is a P wave **taller** than 2.5 mm (2.5 little boxes).*

In *left atrial enlargement* (*LAE*), the P wave becomes wider and often notched (Figure 1–3C). Depolarization of the LA is delayed, resulting in a wider P wave. If the contributions of the RA and the LA are widely separated, a notch may be seen between them. The overall voltage of the P wave generally does not increase, since the contributions of the two atria overlap less.

*Standard criterion for LAE in lead II is a P wave that is **wider** than 0.10s (2.5 little boxes).*

B. P Waves in Lead V1

In lead V1, P waves may normally be biphasic (Figure 3–2). The RA is anterior to the LA, and the depolarization of the RA comes toward V1, resulting in a positive deflection for the first half of the P wave. The depolarization of the LA goes away from V1, resulting in a negative deflection for the second half of the P wave.

If one of the atria are enlarged, then the contribution of that atrium will predominate. Thus, *in RAE, the first part of the biphasic*

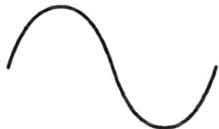

Lead V1: Normal P wave morphology

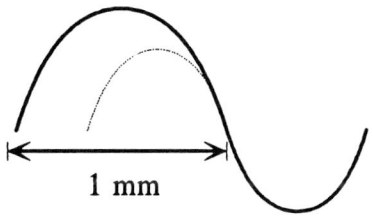

Lead V1: Right atrial enlargement

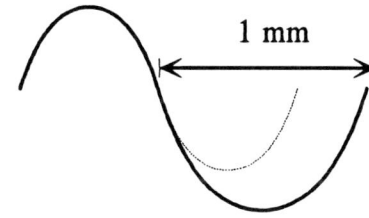

Lead V1: Left atrial enlargement

FIGURE 3–2. P wave morphology in lead V1.

P wave is larger, and *in LAE, the second part of the biphasic P wave is larger.*

*Standard criterion for atrial enlargement in lead V1 is that the appropriate half of the P wave is **greater than 1 mm wide.***

C. Summary of Changes in Atrial Enlargement

The changes associated with atrial enlargement are shown in Figure 3–3.

Right atrial enlargement

Tall, peaked P waves in lead II (greater than 2.5 mm)

Biphasic P wave in lead V1, first part bigger

Occurs in congenital heart disease, in tricuspid valve disease, and in chronic lung disease

Left atrial enlargement

Wide, notched P wave in lead II (wider than 2.5 mm), reflecting interatrial conduction defect

Biphasic P wave in lead V1, second part bigger

Occurs in mitral valve disease, may occur acutely with papillary muscle dysfunction

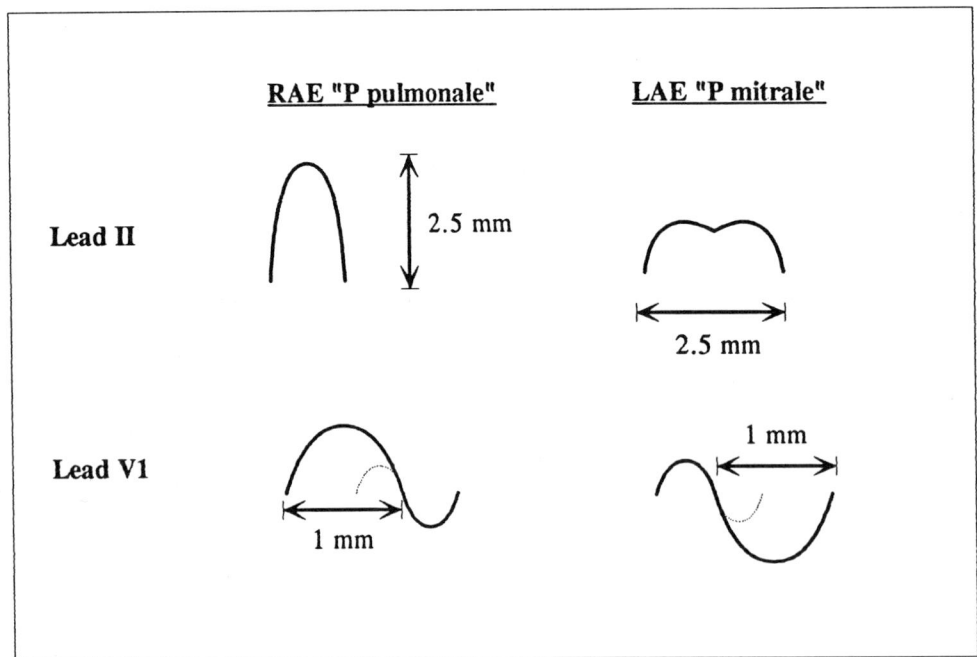

FIGURE 3–3. Summary of changes in atrial enlargement.

III. VENTRICULAR HYPERTROPHY

A. Left Ventricular Hypertrophy (LVH)

Recall how the QRS complex is derived in V1 and V6. The majority of the contribution to the QRS complex is from the left ventricle, so when there is LVH, the voltage of the QRS complex is bigger (Figure 3–4).

There are various criteria for LVH. We will consider three of the most commonly used criteria:

1. **Sokolow and Lyon's voltage criterion:** *If the sum of the S wave in V1 and the R wave in V5 or V6 (whichever is taller) exceeds 35 mm (35 little boxes), then LVH is present.*

This is the criterion that we will generally use in this book. It applies to people over age 35, since younger people often normally have tall QRS voltage without LVH.

2. **aVL voltage criterion:** *If the voltage in lead aVL is over 11 mm (11 little boxes), then LVH is present.*

3. **Estes scoring system:** In addition to voltage, Estes system considers other signs of LVH. *Points* are given for certain findings; of a possible 13 points, if 4 are present, there is *probable* LVH, and if 5 are present, *LVH is present* (see Figure 3–5).

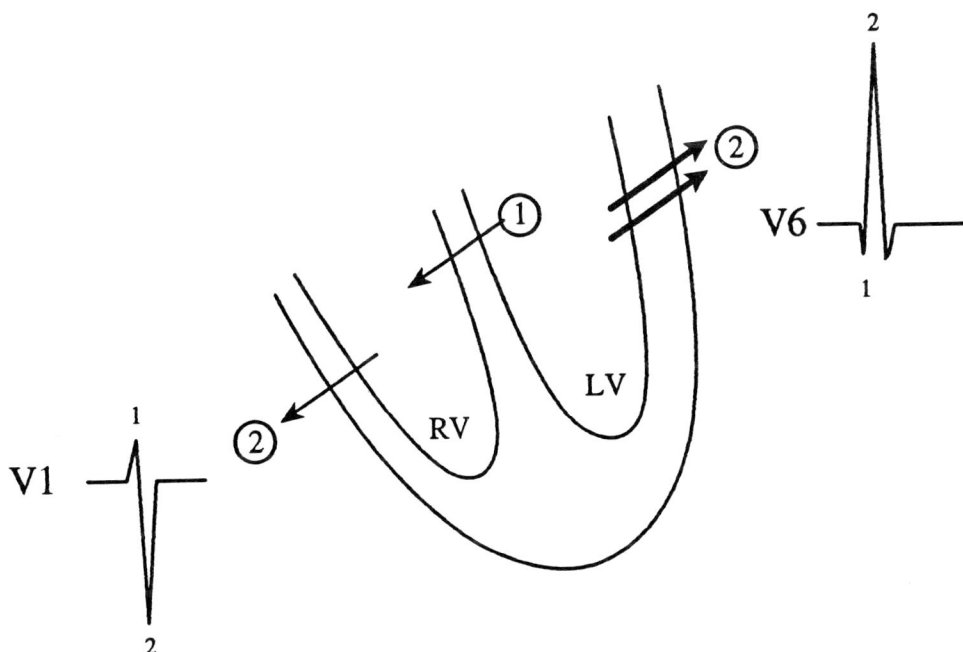

FIGURE 3–4. Contribution of the LV to the QRS voltage.

A.	Voltage criteria: R or S wave in any limb lead >20 mm, or S in V1, V2, or V3 >25 mm, or R wave in V4, V5, or V6 >25 mm	3 points
B.	ST-segment depression pattern, if no digitalis If digitalis is present, pattern must be "typical," and only 1 point is given.	3 points
C.	Axis deviation to the left, more than −15 degrees	2 points
D.	QRS duration greater than 0.09s	1 point
E.	Intrinsicoid deflection, the time from beginning of QRS to its peak, takes 0.04s (one little box) or more	1 point
F.	Left atrial enlargement change in V1, meaning second part of V1 negative and at least 1 mm (one little box) wide	3 points

FIGURE 3–5. Estes' scoring system for LVH.

LVH occurs in hypertension, aortic stenosis, aortic insufficiency, and hypertrophic cardiomyopathy.

B. Right Ventricular Hypertrophy (RVH)

The RV is usually overshadowed by the LV in generating the QRS complex. Thus it may be difficult to tell RVH on an electrocardiogram unless it is marked.

There are two major findings typical of RVH; for reliable diagnosis of RVH, **both** have to be satisfied:

1. *Right axis deviation greater than 100 degrees*
2. *R/S ratio greater than 1 in lead V1 or R/S ratio less than 1 in V6*

RVH occurs with congenital heart disease, mitral stenosis, tricuspid insufficiency, and chronic lung disease and/or cor pulmonale.

C. Strain Pattern

In *systolic overload* of a ventricle, as occurs in aortic stenosis or hypertension, there are ST-T wave changes that look like myocardial ischemia (ST depression). Because these may occur without coronary disease, they are not referred to as ischemia, but rather as a *strain pattern* or *secondary changes of ventricular hypertrophy*. With *diastolic overload*, as in aortic insufficiency, these changes are not present.

Strain patterns may be seen with both LVH and RVH.

IV. SUMMARY

For each electrocardiogram, you should now be able to

1. Determine the rate.
2. Calculate the PR interval, the QRS duration, and the QT interval.
3. Determine the QRS axis.
4. Look at the R-wave progression and tell if it is normal, poor, or "too good."
5. *Look at the P waves in leads II and V1 for evidence of left atrial enlargement (LAE) or right atrial enlargement (RAE).*
6. *Look at the QRS complex for evidence of left ventricular hypertrophy (LVH) or right ventricular hypertrophy (RVH).*

Chapter 4

BUNDLE BRANCH BLOCKS AND HEMIBLOCKS

I. INTRODUCTION

This chapter examines the conduction system of the heart and the normal sequence of activation of the heart, as well as the effects of blocks in this normal activation.

After completing this chapter, you will be able to

1. Examine the QRS duration for evidence of a bundle-branch block; if there is, look in lead V1 to determine if it is a left bundle-branch block (LBBB) or a right bundle-branch block (RBBB).
2. Examine the electrical axis and the QRS morphology to decide if there is evidence for left anterior hemiblock or left posterior hemiblock.

II. NORMAL ACTIVATION OF THE HEART

In normal electrical activation of the heart, the atria depolarize first and then the ventricles. Signals from the *sinoatrial node (SA node*, also called the *sinus node*) depolarize the atria, giving rise to P waves. The electrical impulse then reaches the *atrioventricular node (AV node)*. The signal then goes from the AV node down special conducting system tissue and causes depolarization of the left and right ventricles, giving rise to the QRS complex.

Figure 4–1 is a diagram of the normal conduction system of the heart.

22 □ SECTION I: SYSTEMATIC APPROACH TO ECGs

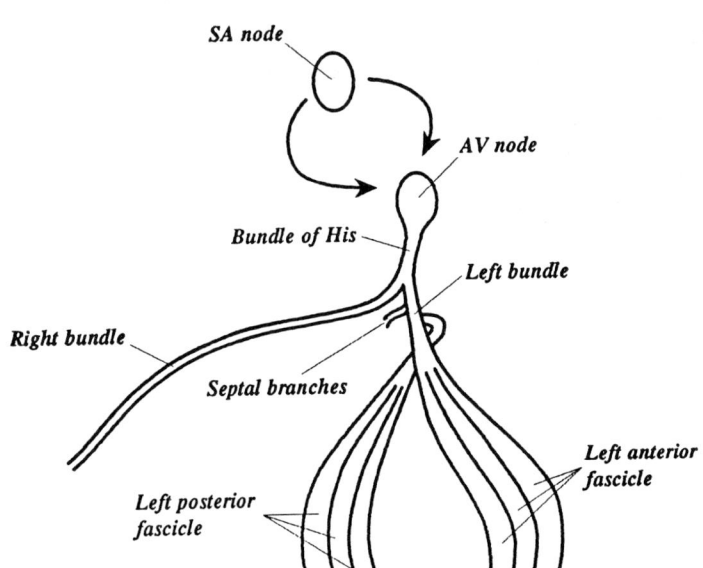

FIGURE 4–1. Conduction system of the heart.

The specialized conduction tissue in the ventricles is called the *His-Purkinje system*. It consists of the *bundle of His*, which separates into the *left and right bundles*.

The His-Purkinje system conducts electrical impulses quickly and gives rise to a narrow, sharp QRS complex. In contrast, when electrical impulses travel through the ventricular muscle tissue itself, the QRS complex is wide and blurred. This may occur if there is a problem with conduction down the His-Purkinje system, called a *bundle-branch block*. It also occurs if there is a premature ventricular beat.

Normally, the duration of the QRS complex is less than 0.12s (3 little boxes). If the QRS duration is prolonged to 0.12s or greater, there is a *bundle-branch block*. If it is 0.10 to 0.12s, there is an *incomplete bundle-branch block*, or an *intraventricular conduction delay (IVCD)*, which can be of the left or right bundle type.

III. PATTERNS OF BUNDLE BRANCH BLOCKS

A. Patterns

The patterns for left and right bundle-branch blocks are shown in Figure 4–2. The most useful leads to look at are V1 and V6.

In left bundle-branch block (LBBB), there is a large QS wave (downward component) in V1.

In right bundle-branch block (RBBB), the first part of the QRS is normal. In V1, there is a large RSR′ complex.

B. Normal QRS Complex

Recall how the QRS complex is derived normally in leads V1 and V6. The steps in ventricular activation are as follows:

1. The septum depolarizes first. Notice from Figure 4–1 that the left bundle normally gives branches to the septum, so septal depolarization occurs from *left to right*. This causes a small upstroke in V1 and a small downstroke in V6 (see Figure 4–3).
2. The right ventricle and the left ventricle depolarize simultaneously, causing opposite effects on the QRS complex. Because the mass of the left ventricle is much greater than the right ventricle, its contribution outweighs that of the right ventricle.

Thus, in lead V1, there is a large downstroke, caused by left ventricular activation away from V1. Similarly, in lead V6, there is a large upstroke, caused by left ventricular activation toward V6.

CHAPTER 4: BUNDLE BRANCH BLOCKS AND HEMIBLOCKS   23

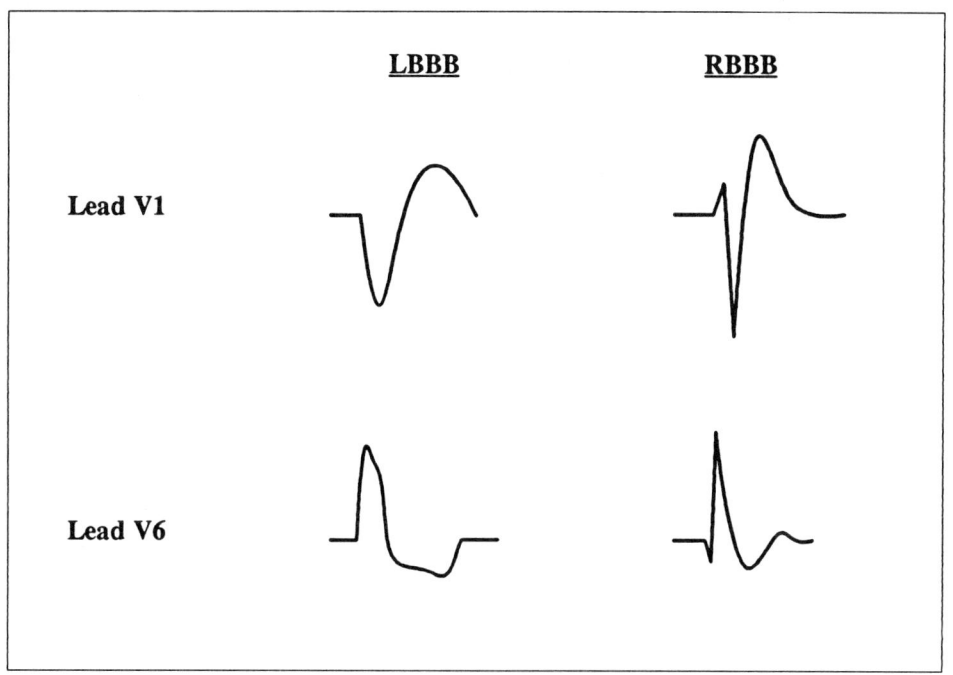

FIGURE 4–2. Patterns of bundle branch blocks in leads V1 and V6.

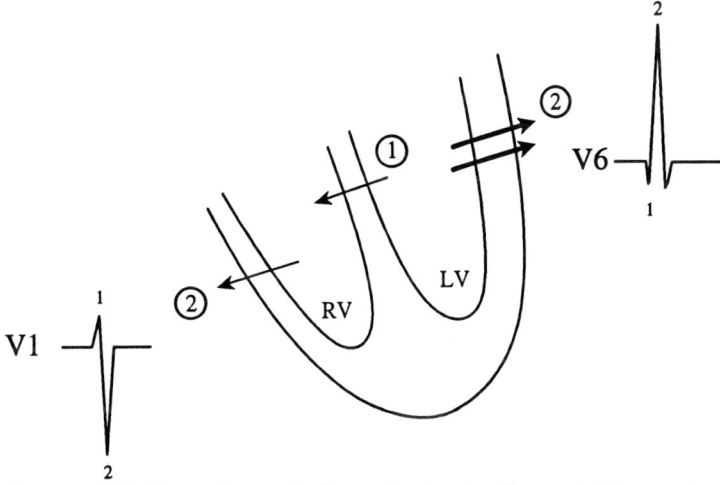

FIGURE 4–3. Normal ventricular activation leading to QRS complex.

C. Left Bundle-Branch Block

Now let's consider what happens in *left bundle-branch block*. Conduction down the left bundle is blocked, so depolarization of the septum and the left ventricle occurs via electrical impulses that travel through the ventricular muscle tissue. This will take longer, meaning that the QRS will be widened.

The steps of ventricular activation are as follows (see Figure 4–4):

1. The septum still depolarizes first, but because the left bundle is blocked, it does so from *right to left*. Septal depolarization is also delayed, so it overlaps with right ventricular depolarization. Septal depolarization goes away from V1, causing a downstroke in that lead. Similarly, septal depolarization goes toward V6, causing an upstroke in that lead.
2. The right ventricle then depolarizes. This is partially masked by septal depolarization, which goes in the opposite direction. If it is not totally masked, there may be a small upstroke in V1 and a small downstroke in V6.
3. The left ventricle depolarizes last, causing a large negative deflection in V1 and a large positive deflection in V6. Because the impulse travels through ventricular muscle tissue, the QRS is wide.

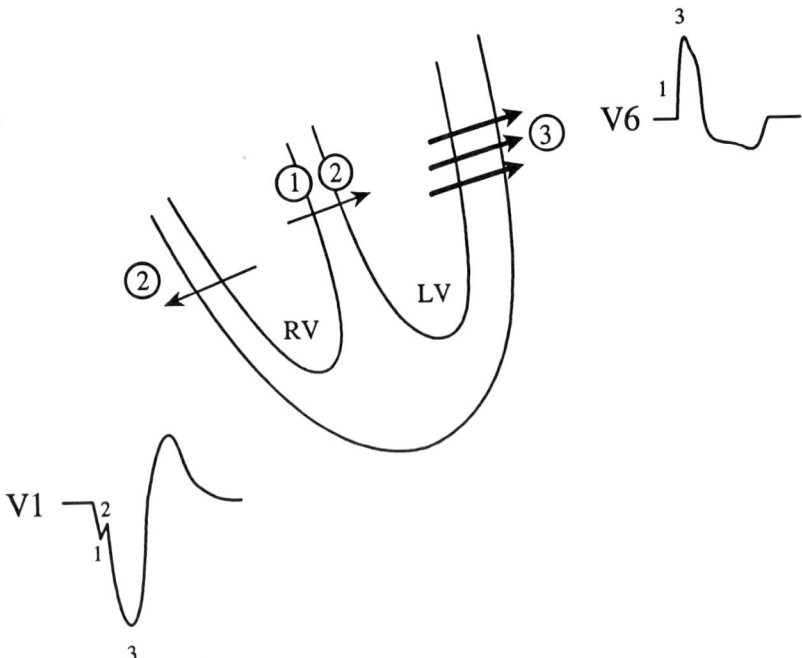

FIGURE 4–4. Ventricular activation in left bundle branch block.

CHAPTER 4: BUNDLE BRANCH BLOCKS AND HEMIBLOCKS 23

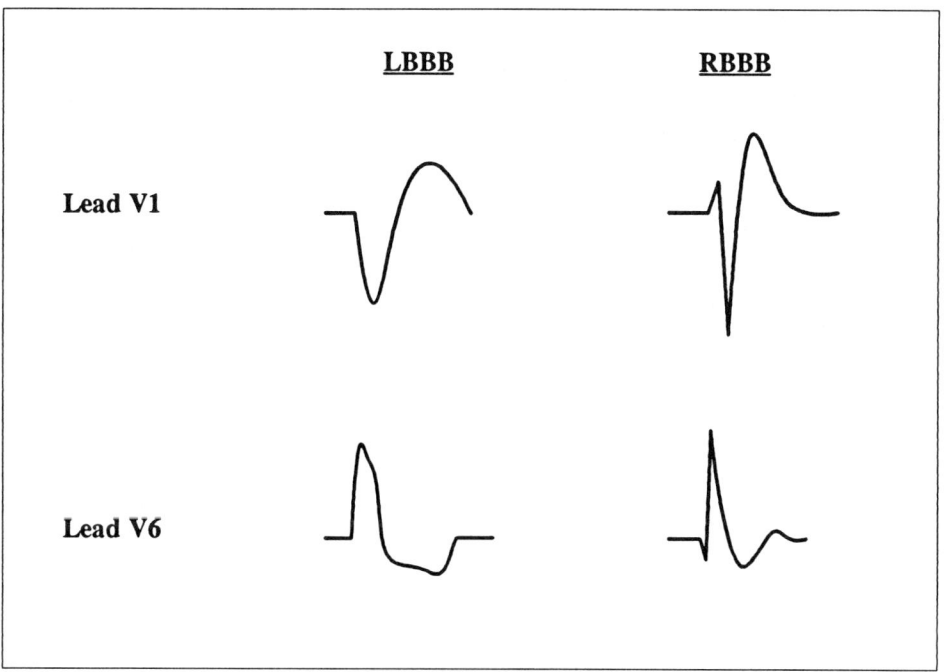

FIGURE 4–2. Patterns of bundle branch blocks in leads V1 and V6.

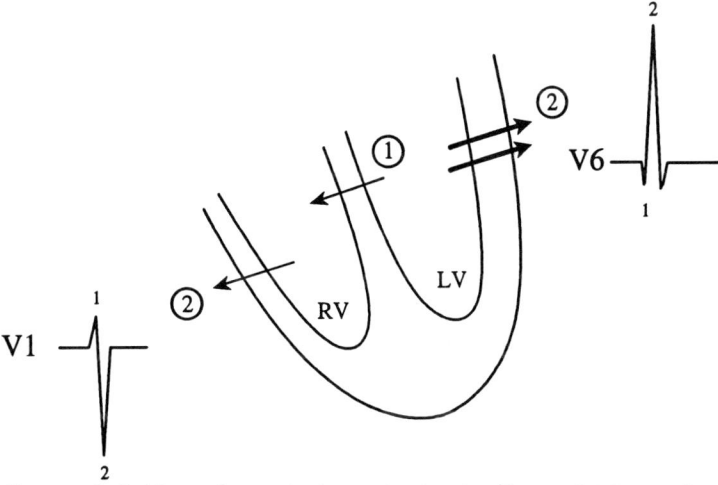

FIGURE 4–3. Normal ventricular activation leading to QRS complex.

C. Left Bundle-Branch Block

Now let's consider what happens in *left bundle-branch block*. Conduction down the left bundle is blocked, so depolarization of the septum and the left ventricle occurs via electrical impulses that travel through the ventricular muscle tissue. This will take longer, meaning that the QRS will be widened.

The steps of ventricular activation are as follows (see Figure 4–4):

1. The septum still depolarizes first, but because the left bundle is blocked, it does so from *right to left*. Septal depolarization is also delayed, so it overlaps with right ventricular depolarization. Septal depolarization goes away from V1, causing a downstroke in that lead. Similarly, septal depolarization goes toward V6, causing an upstroke in that lead.
2. The right ventricle then depolarizes. This is partially masked by septal depolarization, which goes in the opposite direction. If it is not totally masked, there may be a small upstroke in V1 and a small downstroke in V6.
3. The left ventricle depolarizes last, causing a large negative deflection in V1 and a large positive deflection in V6. Because the impulse travels through ventricular muscle tissue, the QRS is wide.

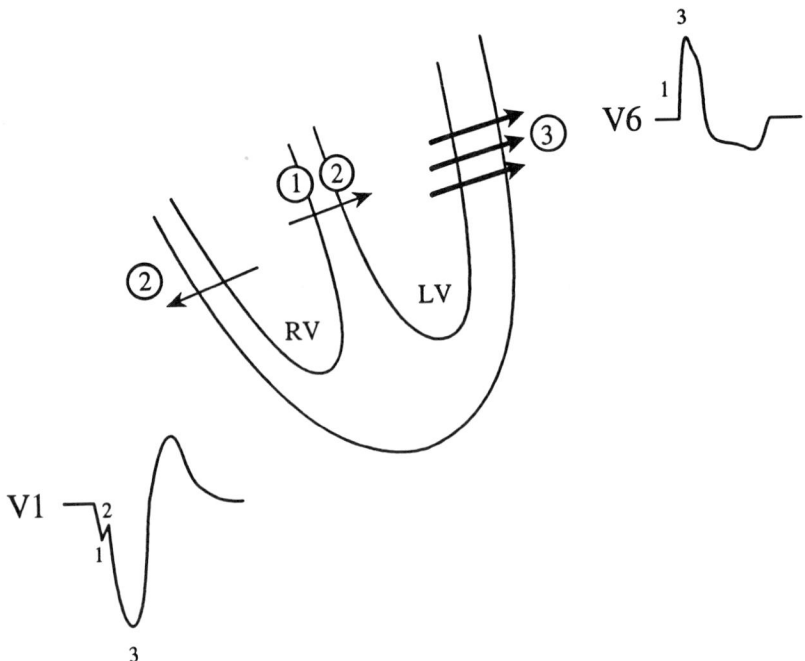

FIGURE 4–4. Ventricular activation in left bundle branch block.

D. Right Bundle-Branch Block

In *right bundle-branch block*, the sequence of ventricular activation is again different (see Figure 4–5):

1. The septum depolarizes normally, from left to right. This leads to a small upstroke in V1 and a small downstroke in V6.
2. The left ventricle depolarizes normally, leading to a large downstroke in V1 and a large upstroke in V6. Because the left ventricle normally contributes most of the voltage to the QRS, the absence of the right ventricular contribution does have a great effect. Notice that the first part of the QRS complex seems quite normal so far.
3. Finally, the right ventricle depolarizes, but it does so through electrical impulses that travel through ventricular muscle. This leads to a wide latter part of the QRS that has a large upstroke in V1 and a large downstroke in V6.

Thus, in lead V1, RBBB gives rise to an RSR′. Note, however, that the first part of the QRS complex is normal in RBBB.

E. Secondary Changes

In bundle-branch block, repolarization as well as depolarization is abnormal. The T waves, which represent repolarization of the ventricles, go in the opposite direction to the main QRS complex. These are called *secondary ST-T wave abnormalities* because they are part of the changes expected from the bundle-branch block alone.

In LBBB, you cannot read ischemia or infarction, since the beginning of the QRS is affected. In RBBB, the first part of the QRS complex is largely normal, so Q waves can be read.

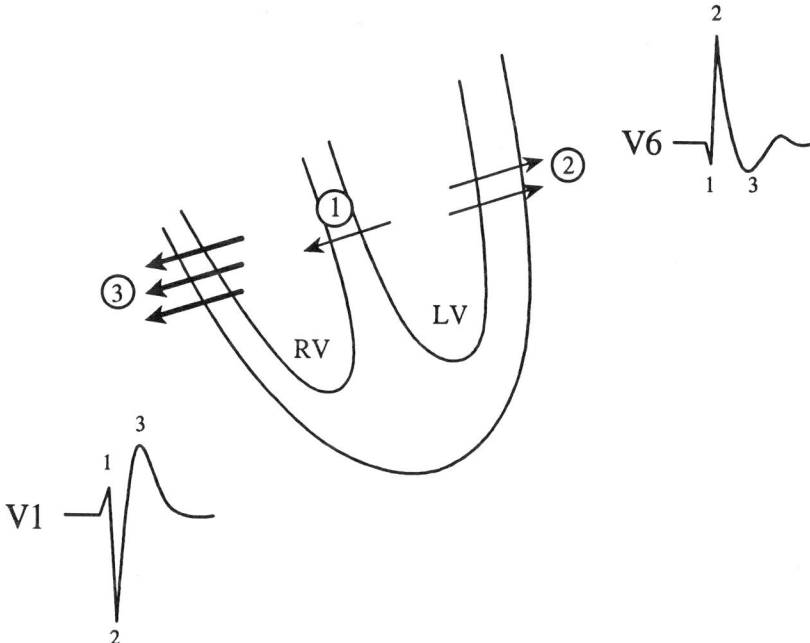

FIGURE 4–5. Ventricular activation in right bundle branch block.

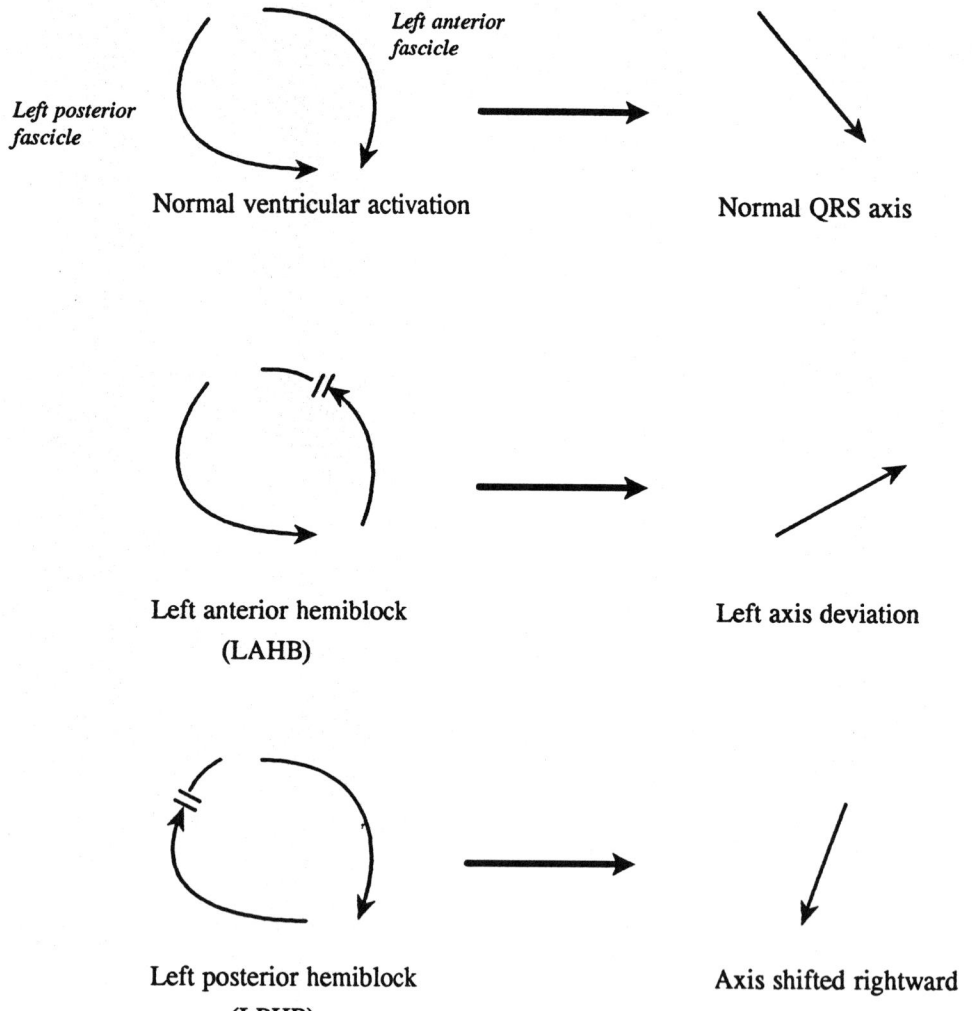

FIGURE 4–6. Left anterior and posterior hemiblocks.

IV. HEMIBLOCKS

The left bundle branch divides into the anterior and posterior fascicles, which then spread throughout the left ventricle. The anterior fascicle is also superior, and the posterior fascicle is also inferior (see Figure 4–1).

If conduction down one of the fascicles is blocked, the depolarization travels down the other fascicle and then passes back over the blocked fascicle. Because the electrical impulse still travels through conduction tissue, there is not much QRS prolongation. However, the *direction* of the impulse is different, and the axis of the QRS will be changed.

Normally, conduction down both anterior and posterior fascicles results in a net QRS axis in the normal range (see Figure 4–6).

In *left anterior hemiblock (LAHB)*, conduction goes down the posterior fascicle normally, but not the anterior fascicle. The impulse travels back over the anterior fascicle, resulting in a shift of the axis to the left, usually to more than −30 degrees. In the absence of LBBB or LVH, LAD more than −30 degrees suggests LAHB (see Figure 4–6).

In *left posterior hemiblock (LPHB)*, the axis is shifted more to the right, but it may still be in the normal quadrant. You need to compare serial ECG tracings unless the axis is clearly abnormally to the right. Also, you must decide that the RAD is not due to RVH (see Figure 4–6).

In LBBB, neither fascicle is used, so you cannot diagnose LAHB or LPHB. LBBB may be associated with left axis deviation, in which case one would call "LBBB with LAD."

In RBBB, you can diagnose hemiblocks in the remaining left bundle branch. Instead of looking at the entire QRS complex, you should look at the first 0.04s, which reflects the left ventricular activation. The eye does this intuitively.

V. SUMMARY

Let's incorporate the identification of bundle-branch blocks and hemiblocks into our systematic approach. For each electrocardiogram, you should now be able to

1. Determine the rate and whether the rhythm is regular.
2. Calculate the PR interval, the QRS duration, and the QT interval.
   A prolonged QRS duration tells you conduction is abnormal. If the QRS is 0.10 to 0.12s, there is an incomplete bundle-branch block, an IVCD. If the QRS duration is 0.12s or greater, there is a bundle-branch block.
   Look in lead V1: If there is a large QS complex, it is a left bundle-branch block. If there is an RSR', it is a right bundle-branch block.
3. Determine the QRS axis.
   If there is LAD, in the absence of LBBB or LVH, you can call LAD consistent with left anterior hemiblock.
   If there is RAD, in the absence of criteria for RVH, you can call left posterior hemiblock. If the axis shifts significantly to the right, you should also suspect left posterior hemiblock.
4. Look at the P waves in leads II and V1 for evidence of left atrial enlargement (LAE) or right atrial enlargement (RAE).
5. Look at the R wave progression and tell if it is normal, poor, or "too good."
6. Look at the QRS complex for evidence of left ventricular hypertrophy (LVH) and right ventricular hypertrophy (RVH).

Chapter 5

ISCHEMIA AND INFARCTION

I. INTRODUCTION

This chapter describes the anatomic distribution of blood supply to the heart and how different areas are reflected in groups of ECG leads. The changes seen in myocardial infarction and ischemia are described.

After completing this chapter, you will be able to

1. Examine the ECG for Q waves, R-wave progression, ST-segment changes, and T-wave changes that may indicate infarction or ischemia.
2. Look at these changes in groups of leads that reflect anatomic areas of the heart and
3. Recognize nonspecific ST-T wave abnormalities.

II. ANATOMIC DISTRIBUTION

A. Coronary Anatomy

The blood supply to the heart is shown in Figure 5–1.

Three major coronary arteries come off the aorta to supply the heart:
    The *left anterior descending artery (LAD)*
    The *left circumflex artery (LCx)*
    The *right coronary artery (RCA)*

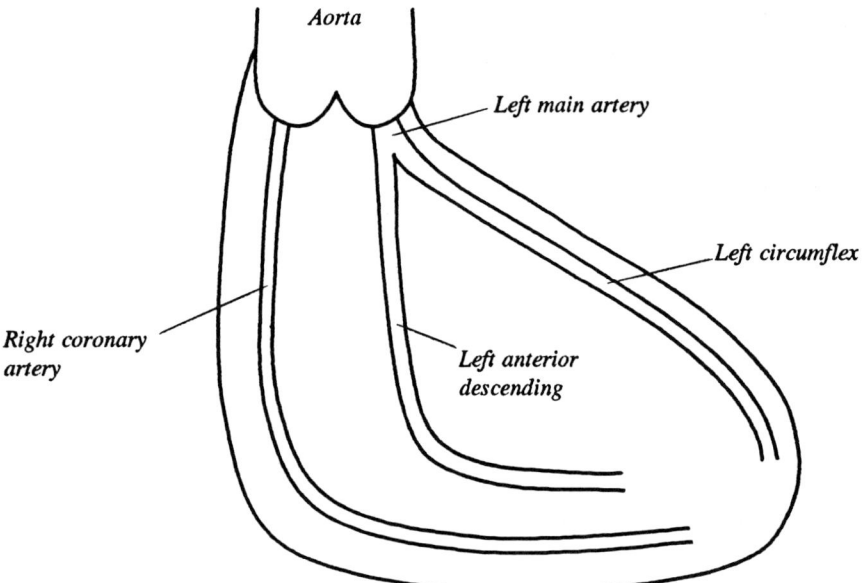

FIGURE 5–1. The major coronary arteries.

The left anterior descending artery and the left circumflex artery usually come off the aorta together, as the *left main artery (LM)*, which then branches. The right coronary artery supplies the inferior and posterior aspects of the heart. The left anterior descending artery supplies the front, or anterior, part of the heart, and the left circumflex artery usually supplies the lateral aspect of the heart. There is great variability in these distributions and the relative size and contributions of these three vessels.

B. Anatomic Groups of Leads

Different leads of the ECG reflect different anatomic areas of the heart. Some typical distributions are listed here, along with the ECG leads that are likely to show changes when these areas are affected:

Anterior	V1–V6
Anteroseptal	V1–V2
Apical	V5–V6
Lateral	I, aVL
Inferior	II, III, aVF
Posterior	Subtle changes in V1 and V2

It is helpful to train your eye to look at these leads as *groups:* II, III, and aVF for inferior changes, V1 through V6 for anterior changes, and I and L for lateral changes (see Figure 5–2).

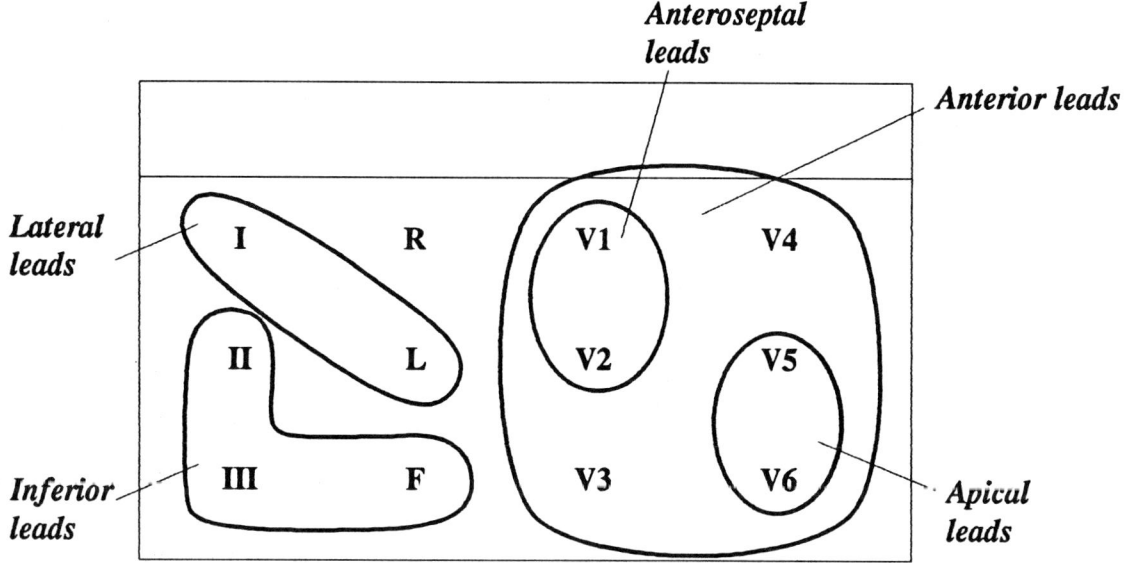

FIGURE 5–2. Anatomic groups of leads.

III. PATTERNS OF ISCHEMIA AND INFARCTION

A. Loss of R Waves

In the precordial leads, V1 through V6, loss of R waves where they were once present may indicate that a myocardial infarction (MI) has occurred. One of the causes of poor R-wave progression is an anteroseptal or anterior MI. Remember, however, that poor R-wave progression also may be caused by lead placement or clockwise rotation.

B. Q Waves

Significant Q waves indicate that myocardial infarction has occurred. To be significant, Q waves must be

1. At least 0.04s (one little box wide), or
2. More than 25% of the R-wave height.

Septal *q* waves may be present in apical and lateral leads I, L, V5, and V6 as a result of septal depolarization away from these leads. They usually do not meet the requirements for significance. An isolated Q wave in lead III does not necessarily indicate infarction, unless there are Q waves in either lead II or lead aVF as well.

Q waves in leads II, III, and aVF suggest an inferior MI; Q waves in the V leads suggest an anterior or an anteroseptal MI.

C. ST-Segment Elevation

ST-segment elevation is a sign of *acute injury* and may indicate that an acute myocardial infarction is occurring.

The causes of ST-segment elevation include
  Acute injury (acute infarction)

Aneurysm formation
Prinzmetal's angina or variant angina due to coronary spasm
Pericarditis
Normal early repolarization

Normal early repolarization is a finding in which the ST segments in the anterior leads, usually V4 through V6, do not fully come down to baseline after the QRS complex before they lead into the T wave. This occurs often in young people and is not a cause for concern. As an example, see Case 3.

D. ST-Segment Depression

Horizontal or downsloping ST-segment depressions are specific for *ischemia* or *subendocardial myocardial infarction (SEMI)*. These changes are often quantitated in terms of the magnitude of the depression (2-mm ST depression, for example).

Upsloping ST-segment depressions are not specific and may be seen in rapid heart rhythms (see Figure 5–3).

E. T-Wave Inversion

T-wave inversion is a repolarization abnormality and is less specific than ST-segment depression. Biphasic T waves have similar implications as inverted T waves.

Like ST-segment depression, T-wave inversions may indicate *ischemia* or *subendocardial myocardial infarction (SEMI)*. They also may indicate *metabolic* or *electrolyte abnormalities*, extensive *neurologic damage* (giving rise to widespread, deep T-wave inversions), or *gallbladder disease* (seen in inferior leads II, III, and aVF).

Even though T-wave changes are not as specific as ST-segment depressions, the inversion of T waves in an anatomic distribution, for instance, in V1 through V6 or in the inferior leads, is of concern. In a patient with known or suspected coronary disease, such T-wave inversions must be taken as a sign of ischemia unless proven otherwise.

F. Reciprocal Changes in Posterior MI

Posterior MIs are difficult to diagnose from Q waves and ST-segment or T-wave changes because no leads are routinely placed over the posterior aspect of the heart. However, the V1 and V2 leads, which reflect changes in the septum, may give important information about the posterior wall.

A Q-wave MI of the posterior wall may result in new tall R waves in V1 and V2 with upright T waves. These are actually Q waves and T-wave inversions of the posterior wall seen upside down in the septal leads; hence they are called *reciprocal changes*.

One of the causes of tall R waves in V1 and V2 (R-wave progression that is "too good") is a posterior MI. When considering this possibility, remember that the posterior wall is usually supplied by the same artery as the inferior wall. Thus, if the

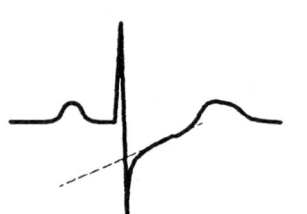 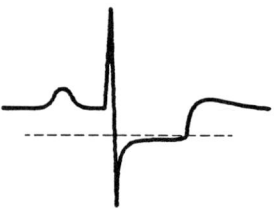 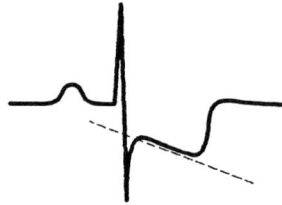

Upsloping ST depression   *Horizontal ST depression*   *Downsloping ST depression*

FIGURE 5–3. Types of ST segment depression.

inferior leads show Q waves, tall R waves in V1 and V2 are more likely to reflect posterior MI.

Another example of reciprocal change is ST-segment depression in V1 and V2 associated with ST-segment elevation in leads II, III, and aVF. The inferior ST-segment elevations point to an acute inferior MI. The anterior ST-segment depressions may reflect *either* acute posterior injury and MI *or* anterior ischemia. Sometimes it is not possible to tell which from the ECG.

IV. EVOLUTION OF INFARCTION

A. Q-Wave Infarction

A classic *Q-wave infarction,* sometimes known as a *transmural infarction,* evolves as follows:

1. Hyperacute T waves — minutes to hours only
2. ST-segment elevation — hours only
3. T wave inversion — hours to days, lasts variably
4. Loss of R waves — hours to days, lasts forever
5. Formation of Q waves — days, lasts for years

An ECG taken minutes after occlusion of a coronary artery may show very peaked T waves, called *hyperacute T waves,* before any other change. As myocardial injury and cell death occur, the ST segments become elevated. Finally, T-wave inversion, loss of R waves, and formation of Q waves occur.

Serial ECGs taken of patients undergoing MI may show these changes over the first few days. However, not all of these steps occur in all infarctions. For example, T-wave inversion may occur without loss of R waves or formation of Q waves.

B. Subendocardial Myocardial Infarction

Non-Q-wave infarctions, sometimes called *subendocardial myocardial infarctions (SEMIs),* may show only ST-segment depression or T-wave inversion. These changes may persist for years. In contrast to a patient who has developed Q waves in a territory from complete coronary occlusion, patients with non-Q-wave MIs may be unstable in that the affected area may be ischemic and may be at risk of further infarction.

Further ischemia in the areas of a SEMI may cause ST-segment depression, ST-segment elevation, further T-wave inversion, or *pseudonormalization* of the T waves, that is, return of inverted T waves to the upright position.

V. NONSPECIFIC ST-T WAVE ABNORMALITIES

The term *nonspecific ST-T wave abnormalities* is probably one of the most frequently used, yet difficult to define, terms in the interpretation of ECGs.

So far we have seen two types of ST-segment and T-wave changes.

First, there are changes that are suggestive of ischemia or infarction in patients with known or suspected coronary artery disease:

Horizontal or downsloping ST depression
ST-segment elevation, and
T-wave inversion

Second, there are ST-segment changes and T-wave changes due to bundle-branch block or ventricular hypertrophy, where the ST segments and T waves are directed opposite to the main direction of the QRS complex. These are secondary changes of bundle-branch block or ventricular hypertrophy and do not necessarily indicate the presence of coronary artery disease.

There is a third group of ST-segment and T-wave changes that are not due to coronary disease nor to bundle-branch block or ventricular hypertrophy. They are collectively called *nonspecific changes* and may include T waves that are shallow, upright or inverted, biphasic, or flattened. Whether to specifically mention them is a matter of judgment. *If the ST segments and T waves do not appear normal but are not clearly ischemic or due to secondary changes, they are nonspecific ST-T wave abnormalities (NSSTTA).*

VI. SUMMARY

For each tracing, you should now be able to

1. Look at leads in *groups* that reflect anatomic distributions:
   II, III, and aVF for inferior changes
   V1 through V6 for anterior changes
   I and L for lateral changes

2. Look for
   Significant Q waves that indicate infarction.
   ST-segment elevation that may indicate acute injury and infarction.
   Horizontal or downsloping ST-segment depression that may indicate ischemia or SEMI.
   T-wave inversions that may indicate ischemia, SEMI, or be nonspecific.

3. Decide if there are ST-segment and T-wave abnormalities that are not specific for coronary artery disease or due to secondary changes of bundle-branch block or ventricular hypertrophy, and call these NSSTTA.

In the next chapter we will quickly review our systematic approach to reading ECGs and incorporate these steps.

Chapter 6

REVIEW OF SYSTEMATIC APPROACH

I. OVERVIEW

The next three chapters cover arrhythmias. At this point, it may be helpful to review the systematic approach that we have developed so far. With the exception of the rhythm, you have mastered all the other topics that are necessary for the interpretation of electrocardiograms.

The steps to our systematic approach are listed in order. The last step of any interpretation is to compare the tracing with the last previous tracing. *This is very important and cannot be overemphasized:* The last line of any interpretation should be either a comparison with the last tracing or a statement that no previous tracings are available.

II. SYSTEMATIC APPROACH TO READING ECGs

1. Determine the *rate* and *rhythm*.
2. Determine the *intervals:*
   If PR < 0.12s, consider Wolff-Parkinson-White syndrome.
   If PR > 0.20s, consider first-degree heart block or higher-grade block.
   If QRS > 0.12s, consider bundle-branch block; look in V1:
   LBBB gives QS.
   RBBB gives RSR′.

3. Determine the *axis*:
   Look in I and aVF to determine which quadrant the axis is in. Find the isoelectric lead and then decide on the axis.
   If LAD (left axis deviation), if there is no LBBB or LVH, call "LAD consistent with left anterior hemiblock."
   If RAD (right axis deviation), consider either left posterior hemiblock or RVH. Remember for RVH, you need RAD and R > S in V1.

4. Look at the *P waves* in leads II and V1 for signs of *atrial enlargement*.

5. Look for signs of *LVH* by voltage. Add the S in V1 to the R in V5 or V6; if it is over 35 mm, call "LVH by voltage."

6. Look for signs of *RVH*. If there is right axis deviation and R > S in V1 or S > R in V6, then you can call "RVH."

7. Look at the *R-wave progression*. R waves should grow from V1 through at least V4. The transition point should be V3 or V4.
   If there is PRWP (poor R-wave progression), consider ASMI, COPD, lead placement, or clockwise rotation (CR).
   If the R-wave progression is too good, consider RVH, RBBB, posterior MI, or counterclockwise rotation (CCR).

8. Look for signs of *ischemia* or *infarction* in anatomic distributions: II, III, aVF, for inferior changes, V1 through V6 for anterior changes, and I and L for lateral changes.
   Look for *Q waves*. An isolated Q wave in lead III is not a cause for concern.
   Look for *ST-segment elevations*, which suggest acute injury (acute MI) or aneurysm.
   Look for *ST-segment depression* or *T-wave inversion*, which suggests ischemia or SEMI.

9. Compare with the last previous tracing. If none is available, state, "No previous tracing available for comparison."

Chapter 7

APPROACH TO ARRHYTHMIAS AND CONDUCTION BLOCKS

I. INTRODUCTION

The arrhythmias are covered in three chapters. This chapter describes the general approach to arrhythmias and begins with AV conduction blocks.

After completing this chapter, you will be able to

1. Look at any cardiac rhythm and begin analysis of the arrhythmia by determining the atrial activity and the origin of the QRS complexes.
2. Recognize the findings of first-degree heart block, Wenkebach and non-Wenkebach second-degree heart block, and complete heart block.

II. APPROACH TO ARRHYTHMIAS

No matter how complex an arrhythmia is, the problem can be unraveled by a systematic approach. With any rhythm, there are two important questions to answer:

1. *What is the atrial activity, and how is it related to the QRS complex?*
2. *Is the QRS complex normal or is it wide?*

A. Atrial Activity

Always look for P waves first. If P waves are found, the atria are being depolarized.

38 □ SECTION I: SYSTEMATIC APPROACH TO ECGs

Next, look for how P waves are related to QRS complexes. A P wave may precede each QRS complex (normal activation), follow a QRS complex (retrograde P waves), have a changing relationship, or be unrelated to the QRS complexes (AV dissociation).

If there are no P waves, the rhythm may be irregular (atrial fibrillation) or regular (junctional or ventricular).

B. QRS Morphology

Determine if the QRS complex is narrow or wide. This will help determine the origin of the complex.

If a QRS complex is *narrow,* the arrhythmia is supraventricular. The complexes must originate in the atria or junctional tissue (AV node and His bundle).

If a QRS complex is *wide,* it may either be (1) *ventricular* or (2) *supraventricular* with aberrant conduction. The simplest case of a QRS complex from a supraventricular source with aberrant conduction is the bundle-branch blocks. In LBBB and RBBB, QRS complexes that are trigerred by normal sinus node activity are wide because of abnormal conduction in the ventricles.

C. Automaticity

Different parts of the heart display different *automaticity,* meaning that they naturally beat on their own at a certain rate. These are called *pacemaker centers.*

Pacemaker Center	Normal Automaticity
Sinoatrial (SA) node	60–100 beats per minute
Junction (AV node and His bundle)	40–50 beats per minute
Ventricular cells	30–40 beats per minute

Normally, the sinoatrial (SA) node, also called the *sinus node,* has the fastest automaticity. The junction and ventricular cells do not normally fire because they receive electrical impulses that originate from the SA node faster than they would fire themselves.

Unexpected beats may be either premature or escape beats. *Premature beats* occur sooner than a normal QRS would have occurred because a focus that normally should not be firing does so. *Escape beats* occur after a pause, when a pacemaker center fires on its own when it has not received an electrical impulse from a faster pacemaker center.

Escape beats do not always occur as expected. In people with arrhythmias, in whom there is a problem with conduction to begin with, the pacemaker centers also may be abnormal.

III. ATRIOVENTRICULAR BLOCKS

A. First-Degree AV Block (Figure 7–1)

Each P wave still precedes a QRS complex, but the PR interval is greater than 0.20s (5 little boxes).

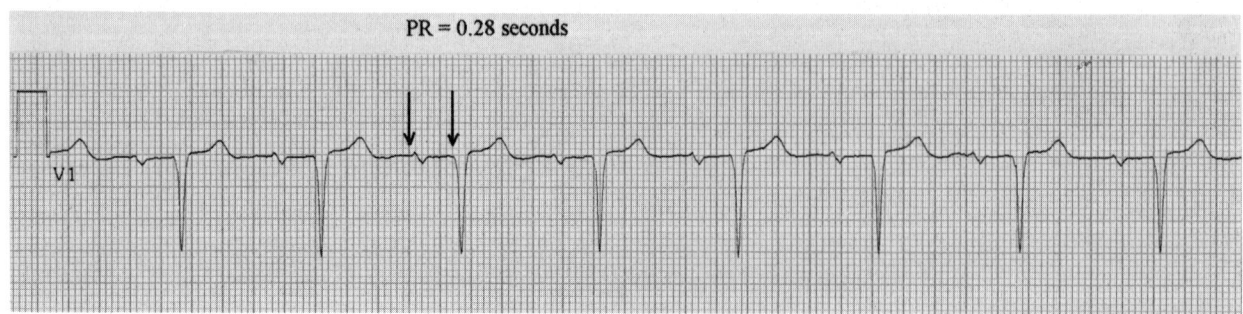

FIGURE 7–1. First degree AV block

First-degree block may be due to drugs that slow AV nodal conduction, ischemia or infarction of the AV node, or disease of the conduction system.

B. Second-Degree Heart Block

P waves occur regularly, but some, not all, P waves are conducted to the ventricles. The ratio of P waves to QRS complexes is often cited; for example, *2:1 block* means that every other P wave is followed by a QRS complex. There are two types, as follows:

Type I block, or Wenkebach block (Figure 7–2)

There is progressive lengthening of the PR interval until there is a dropped beat (a P wave that is not followed by a QRS). The PR interval of the next conducted beat is short again. Look for clustering of beats.

Wenkebach block is often seen in inferior MI and is not as serious as non-Wenkebach second-degree heart block.

Type II block, or non-Wenkebach block (Figure 7–3)

Not all P waves are conducted, but the PR interval of conducted beats is constant. This is a more serious arrhythmia than Wenkebach block and may progress to complete heart block.

Note that it is not possible to tell if a 2:1 second-degree block is Wenkebach type or not. There are no successive PR intervals to show if the PR prolongs or stays constant.

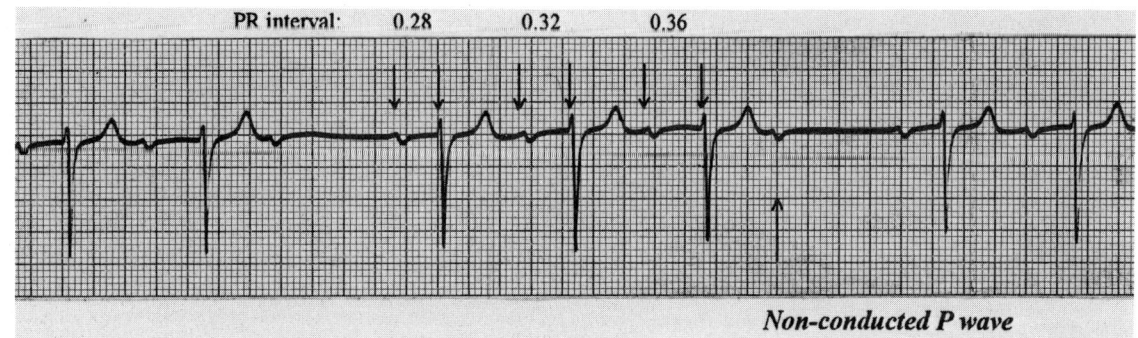

FIGURE 7–2. Second degree heart block: Type I, or Wenkebach block

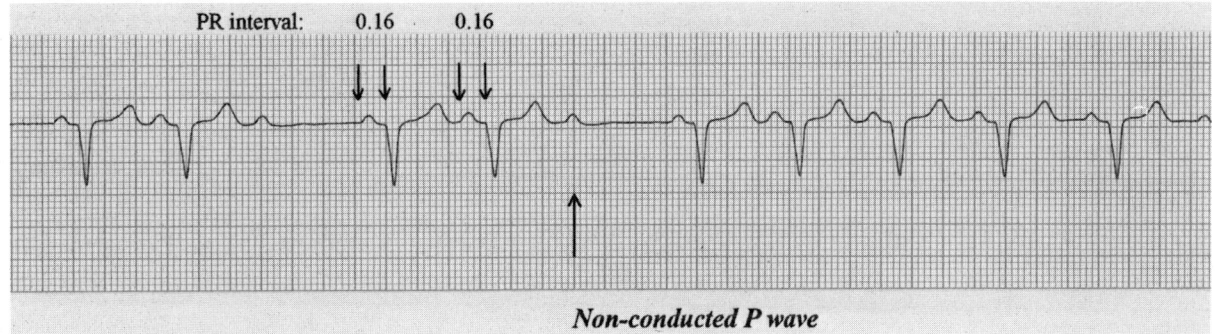

FIGURE 7–3. Second degree heart block: Type II

C. Third-Degree Heart Block (Figure 7–4)

In third-degree block, also called *complete heart block,* there is total absence of AV conduction. P waves and QRS complexes each march independently, with ventricles beating regularly from junctional or ventricular escape. This is a form of AV dissociation.

If the QRS complexes are *narrow,* they must originate from the junctional tissues. If the QRS complexes are *wide,* they must originate from the ventricular cells.

D. AV Dissociation

AV dissociation occurs when the atria and the ventricles beat separately and independently. It is not synonymous with complete heart block because complete heart block is only one of its possible causes. Other causes include either a slowing of the sinus rate or an acceleration of the junctional or ventricular rate so that the junction or ventricles are faster than the sinus node.

These are the causes of AV dissociation:

1. Sinus bradycardia with junctional or ventricular escape
2. Acceleration of subsidiary pacemaker:
   Junctional tachycardia
   Accelerated idioventricular rhythm (AIVR), or
   Ventricular tachycardia (VT)
3. Complete heart block

The major *electrocardiographic* feature of AV dissociation is that the P waves and the QRS complexes each proceed at their own rate, independently of each other. On *physical examination,* two findings are classical for AV dissociation:

1. Cannon A waves—intermittent, large A waves seen in the jugular venous pulse from the right atrium contracting against a closed tricuspid valve.
2. Variable loudness of the S_1—due to closure of the mitral and tricuspid valves from ventricular contraction at varying degrees of atrial contraction

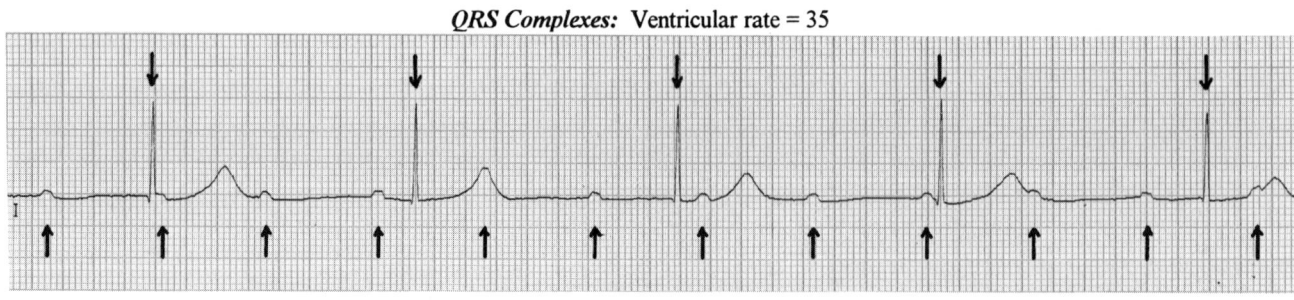

FIGURE 7–4. Third degree AV block; complete heart block with junctional escape

IV. SUMMARY

The analysis of arrhythmias begins with answering two important questions:

1. What is the atrial activity, and how is it related to the QRS complexes?
2. Is the QRS complex wide or narrow?

In AV conduction blocks, the conduction from the atria to the ventricles is abnormal. In first-degree block, all the P waves are conducted, but the PR interval is longer than 0.20s. In second-degree block, some, but not all, P waves are conducted. In third-degree or complete heart block, no P waves are conducted, and the atria and ventricles beat independently.

In addition to complete heart block, the other mechanism for AV dissociation is slowing of the sinus or acceleration of the junctional or ventricular pacemakers so that they are faster than the sinus node.

Chapter 8

SUPRAVENTRICULAR ARRHYTHMIAS

I. INTRODUCTION

This chapter describes supraventricular rhythms, from sinus rhythms to tachyarrhythmias such as atrial fibrillation and atrial flutter. These rhythms give rise to narrow QRS complexes unless there is a bundle-branch block.

After completing this lesson, you will be able to recognize the following rhythms:
  Sinus rhythms (normal sinus rhythm, sinus bradycardia and
    sinus tachycardia)
  Atrial premature beats
  Wandering atrial pacemaker and multifocal atrial tachycardia
  Paroxysmal atrial tachycardia
  Atrial fibrillation
  Atrial flutter
  Junctional rhythm

II. ATRIAL RHYTHMS

A. Sinus Rhythm (Figure 8–1)

The sinus node (SA node) normally depolarizes at a rate between 60 and 100 beats per minute. Sinus rhythm faster than 100 beats per minute is *sinus tachycardia* and slower than 60 beats per minute is *sinus bradycardia*.

The sinus rate usually increases slightly with inspiration, but if

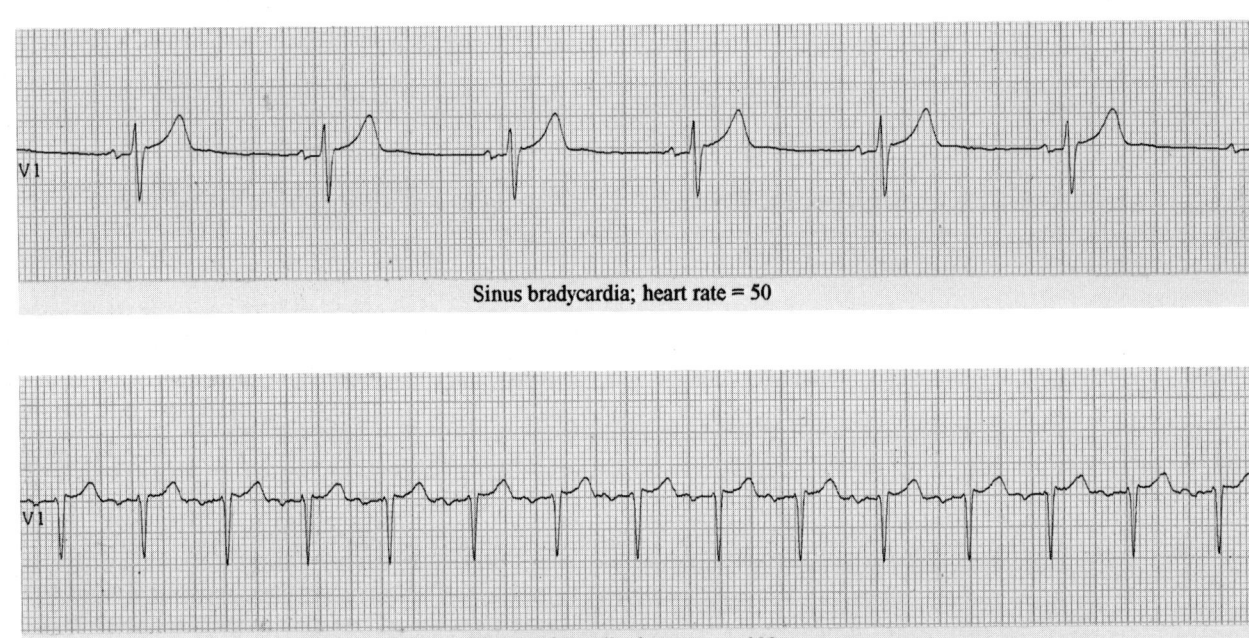

Figure 8-1. Sinus rhythms: sinus bradycardia and sinus tachycardia

the rate varies markedly, one can read sinus arrhythmia instead of normal sinus rhythm.

B. Atrial Premature Beats (Figure 8-2)

Atrial premature beats (APBs) arise from ectopic atrial foci and may lead to a QRS complex that is earlier than expected. Because the atria are depolarized in a different manner, the P-wave morphology will not be the same as a P wave from the sinus node.

APBs are common. If they occur while the AV node is still refractory, they may not be conducted to the ventricles. This results in a pause in the rhythm. In fact, *the most common cause of a pause is a blocked APB*. If there is a pause, look for a blocked APB, which may be buried in the preceding T wave.

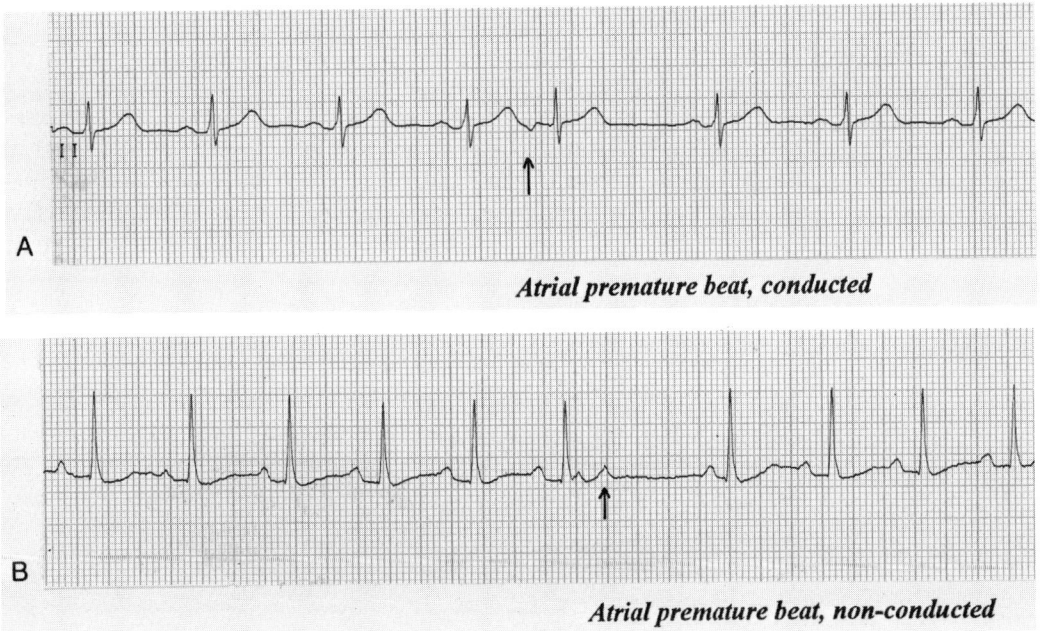

FIGURE 8–2. *A*, Atrial premature beat; *B*, Blocked atrial premature beat

C. Low Atrial Pacemaker (Figure 8–3)

Sometimes there is a pacemaker center in the atrium that fires instead of the sinus node. If this happens, the P-wave morphology will not be normal. An atrial pacemaker low in one of the atria will depolarize the atria upward, resulting in inverted P waves in leads II, III, and aVF.

The other reason for inverted P waves in leads II, III, and aVF is a junctional rhythm where, likewise, the atria are depolarized upward instead of downward.

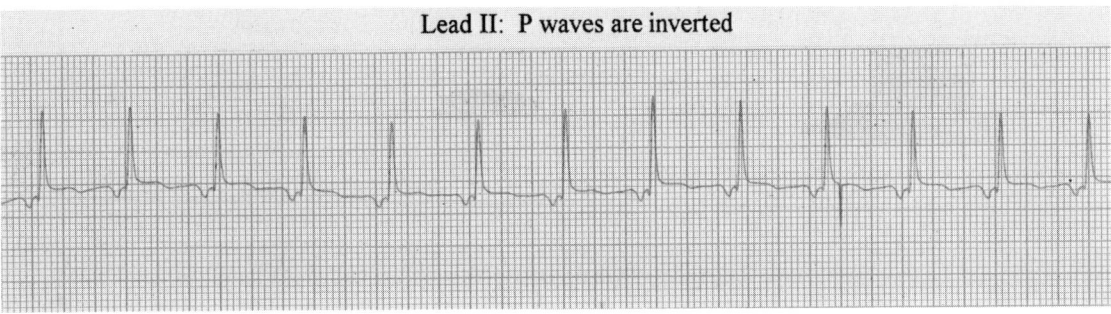

FIGURE 8–3. Low atrial pacemaker (ectopic atrial rhythm)

46 □ SECTION I: SYSTEMATIC APPROACH TO ECGs

D. Wandering Atrial Pacemaker (Figure 8–4)

Wandering atrial pacemaker (WAP) is a rhythm where multiple foci within the atria fire, instead of just the sinus node. The result is an irregular rhythm, usually less than 100 beats per minute. Each atrial pacemaker gives rise to its own distinct P-wave morphology. To make the diagnosis, you should be able to point out at least three different P-wave morphologies. WAP is generally benign.

E. Multifocal Atrial Tachycardia (Figure 8–5)

Multifocal atrial tachycardia (MAT) is similar to wandering atrial pacemaker in that multiple atrial pacemaker foci fire and there are at least three different P-wave morphologies. The rate is usually over 100 beats per minute.

MAT is associated with chronic lung disease and metabolic derangements. Hypoxia, respiratory acidosis, and metabolic alkalosis may all play a part. MAT generally does not deteriorate into worrisome rhythms. MAT itself should not be treated with antiarrhythmics, but rather, the underlying condition should be treated, for example, improving oxygenation, correcting acidosis, and so on.

Because it is an irregular, fast rhythm, MAT is often confused with atrial fibrillation. However, in MAT, clearly recognizable P waves are present. MAT does *not* respond to digoxin.

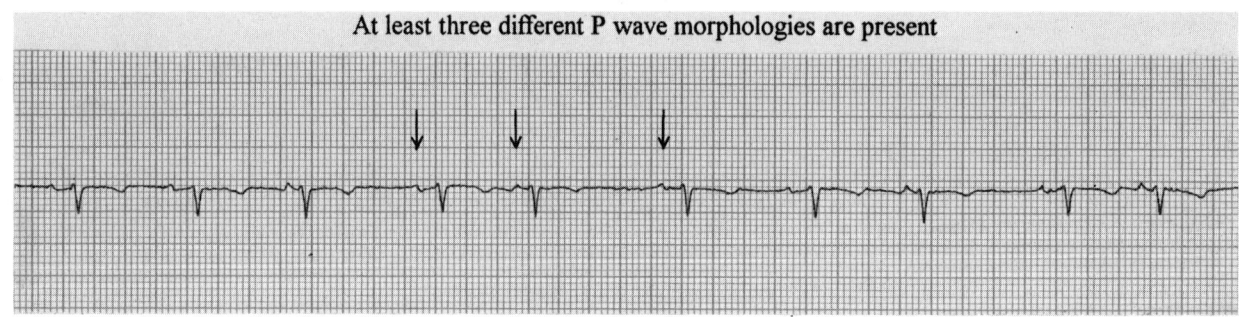

FIGURE 8–4. Wandering atrial pacemaker

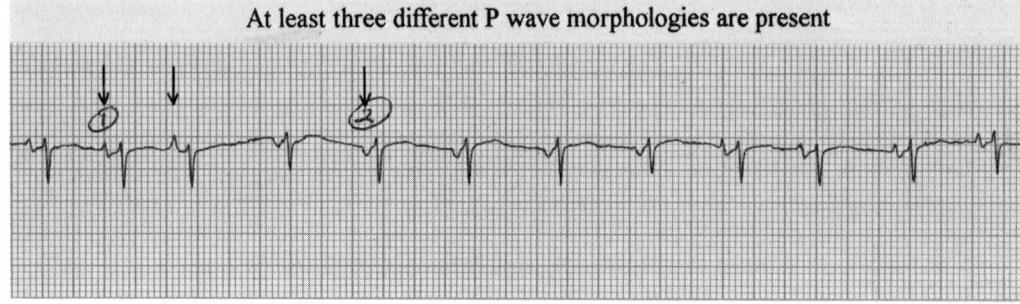

FIGURE 8–5. Multifocal atrial tachycardia

F. Paroxysmal Atrial Tachycardia and Paroxysmal Supraventricular Tachycardia (Figure 8–6)

So far we have dealt with rhythms in which the pacemaker center (sinus node or ectopic atrial foci) gives rise to an impulse that then goes through the AV node to the ventricles.

One common mechanism of tachyarrhythmias in which this normal sequence does not occur is *reentry*. In a reentry mechanism, an impulse travels around in a loop that comes back on itself, resulting in a self-perpetuating cycle.

When the reentry circuit involves the AV node itself, the result is *paroxysmal atrial tachycardia (PAT)*, a term interchangeable with *paroxysmal supraventricular tachycardia (PSVT)*. The hallmarks of PAT are a regular, rapid rhythm, occurring at 150 to 220 beats per minute. PAT is *paroxysmal* in that it can arise suddenly from normal sinus rhythm without warning and may stop suddenly as well.

By virtue of its mechanism, PAT may be interrupted by medications that block or slow conduction through the AV node. When it occurs in digoxin toxicity, PAT is often associated with AV nodal block so that not all the cycles are conducted to the ventricles.

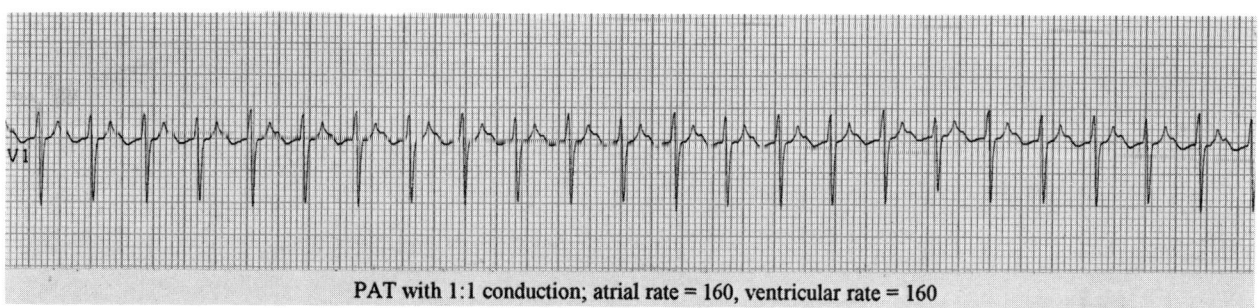

PAT with 1:1 conduction; atrial rate = 160, ventricular rate = 160

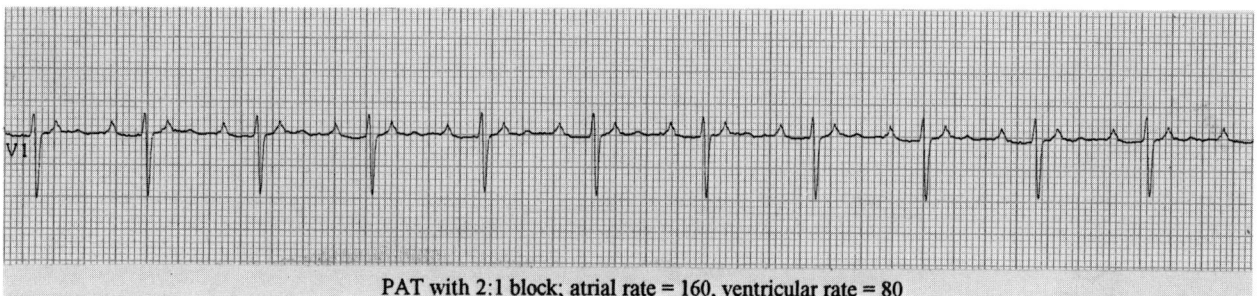

PAT with 2:1 block; atrial rate = 160, ventricular rate = 80

FIGURE 8–6. Paroxysmal atrial tachycardia

G. Atrial Flutter (Figure 8–7)

Another reentry arrhythmia is *atrial flutter*. This time, the reentry circuit does not involve the AV node but is entirely within the atria. The rate of atrial flutter is usually 300 beats per minute. Because the AV node is not able to conduct this fast, there is usually a 2:1 block, so the ventricular rate is 150 beats per minute.

To diagnose atrial flutter, look for sawtooth flutter waves at a rate of 300 beats per minute in inferior leads (II, III, and aVF). When the ventricular rate is exactly 150 beats per minute and regular, always consider atrial flutter.

Atrial flutter occurs with higher degrees of AV block as well, especially in patients with conduction problems or those taking medications that slow AV nodal conduction.

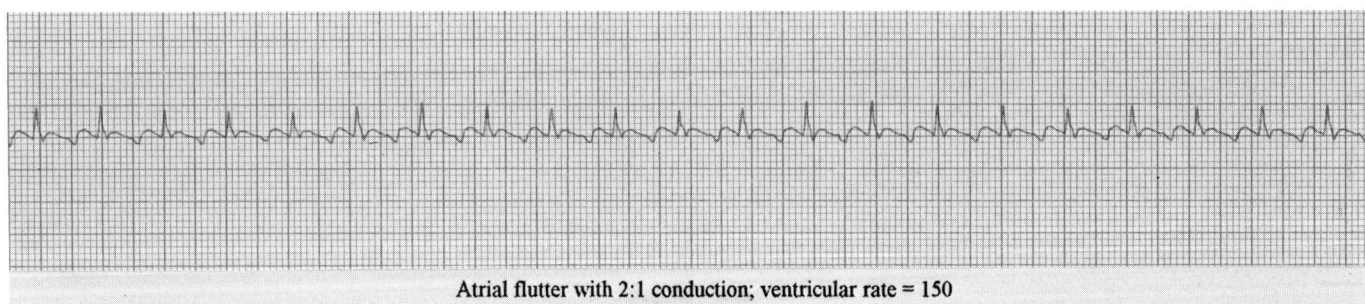

Atrial flutter with 2:1 conduction; ventricular rate = 150

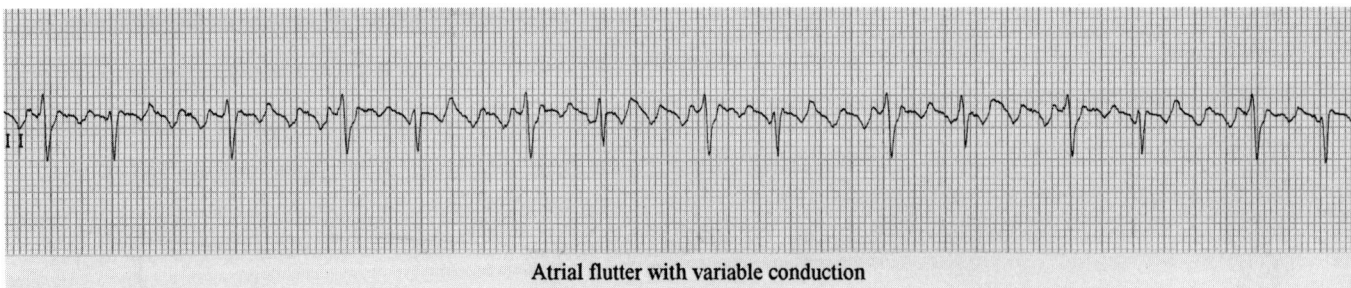

Atrial flutter with variable conduction

FIGURE 8–7. Atrial flutter

H. Atrial Fibrillation (Figure 8–8)

Atrial fibrillation (AF) occurs when atrial depolarization is chaotic, with many different atrial foci bombarding the AV node at rates of 300 to 400 beats per minute. In contrast to PAT and atrial flutter, AF does not have a reentry mechanism and is not regular. The AV node is always partially refractory and only conducts some of the impulses, resulting in a ventricular rate that is totally irregular. The hallmark of AF is an irregular rhythm with no clear P waves.

In describing the rate of AF, the convention is to state that there is atrial fibrillation, with a ventricular reponse that is slow, moderate, or rapid. Less than 60 beats per minute is slow, 60 to 100 beats per minute is moderate, and over 100 beats per minute is rapid. The average ventricular rate is usually not given.

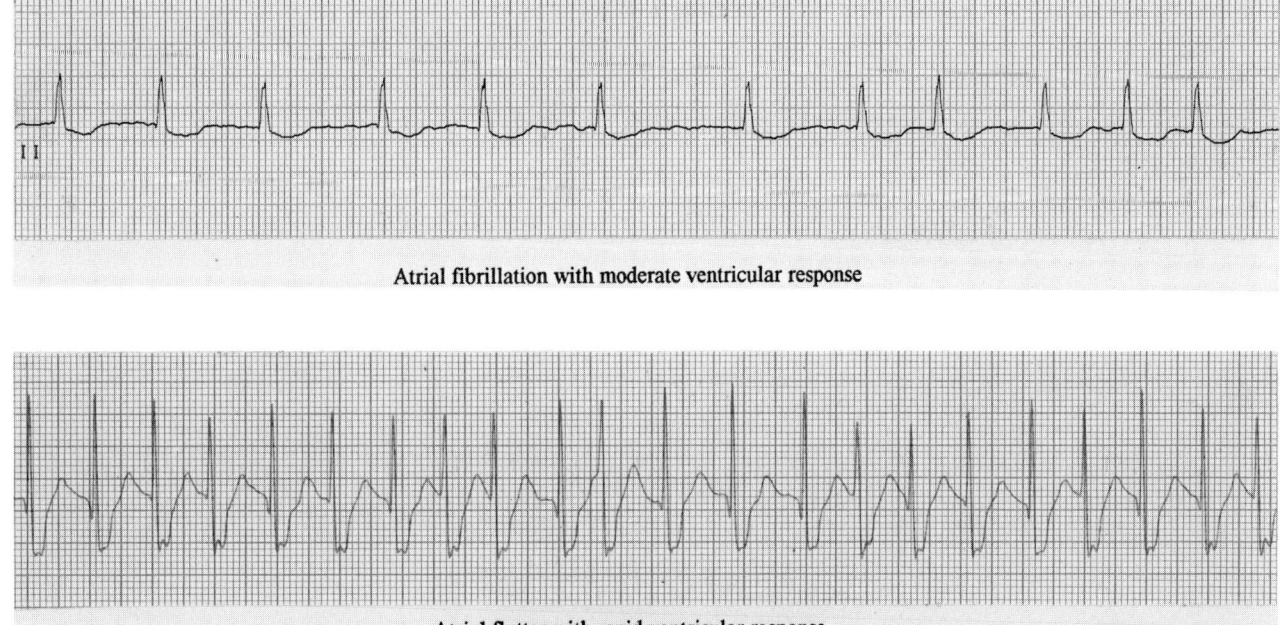

FIGURE 8–8. Atrial fibrillation

III. JUNCTIONAL RHYTHMS

A. Junctional Escape (Figure 8–9)

If there is no sinus rhythm, the pacemaker in the junctional tissues will beat at a rate of 40 to 50 beats per minute. This is *junctional escape,* not tachycardia, since it occurs at the normal rate for the junction. This may happen in sinus arrest (absence of atrial activity) or marked sinus bradycardia.

B. Junctional Tachycardia (Figure 8–10)

Junctional tachycardia occurs when the pacemaker in the junctional tissues (AV node and His bundle) depolarizes spontaneously, not at a rate of 40 to 50 beats per minute, but at faster rates of 100 to 180 beats per minute. The sinus node does not fire because the rate is already fast enough.

The QRS complexes are narrow, and the rhythm is regular. There may be no P waves, or there may be inverted, retrograde P waves in leads II, III, and aVF, which result from depolarization of the atria from the junction upward.

Junctional tachycardia occurs because the junctional tissues are irritated. Causes of junctional tachycardia include:
Ischemia
Digitalis intoxication
Mitral valve edema, often following cardiac surgery
Myocarditis/endocarditis

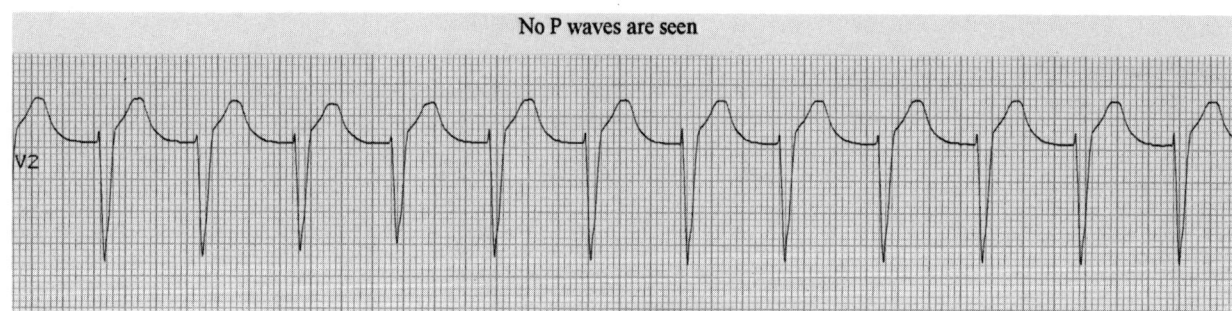

FIGURE 8–9. Junctional tachycardia

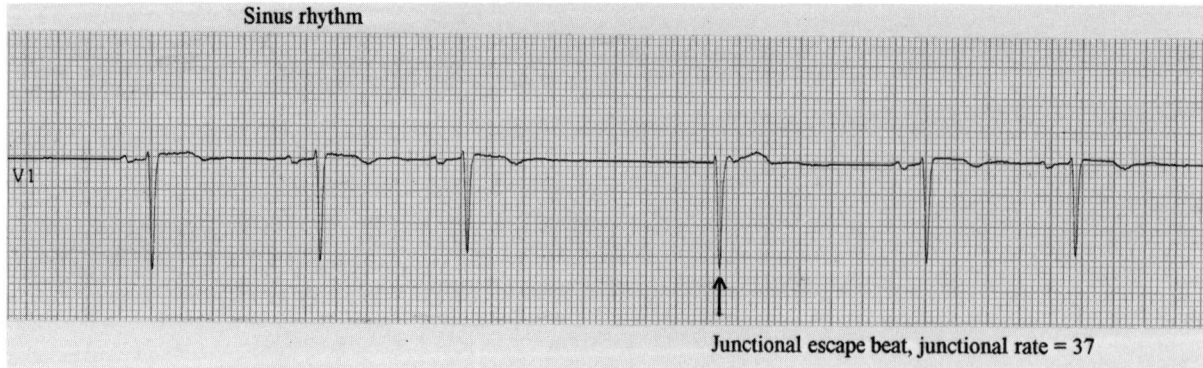

FIGURE 8–10. Sinus rhythm with a pause followed by junctional escape

IV. SUMMARY

Supraventricular rhythms may arise in the sinus node, ectopic atrial foci, or the junctional tissues. They give rise to narrow QRS complexes unless there is a bundle-branch block.

Two regular, rapid rhythms involve a reentry mechanism: PAT/PSVT, where the AV node is part of the reentry circuit, and atrial flutter, where the reentry circuit is entirely within the atria.

Irregular rhythms include atrial fibrillation, where there are no discernible P waves, and WAP or MAT, where there are at least three different P-wave morphologies.

The most common cause of a pause is a blocked atrial premature beat, which is sometimes hidden within the preceding T wave.

Chapter 9

VENTRICULAR ARRHYTHMIAS AND ABERRANCY

I. INTRODUCTION

One of the two important questions to ask with any arrhythmia is whether the QRS complex is narrow or wide. If the QRS complex is *narrow*, it must have originated from the sinus node, atria, or junctional tissues. This chapter describes the rhythms in which the QRS complex is *wide*. These are ventricular rhythms and supraventricular rhythms where there is aberrant conduction.

After completing this chapter, you will be able to

1. Recognize premature ventricular complexes (PVCs), ventricular tachycardia (VT), and ventricular fibrillation.
2. Know the properties of aberrantly conducted beats.

II. VENTRICULAR ARRHYTHMIAS

A. Ventricular Ectopic Activity (VEA) (Figure 9–1)

Foci within the ventricles normally have an intrinsic pacemaker rate of 30 to 40 beats per minute. However, they may fire prematurely, leading to *premature ventricular complexes (PVCs)* (see Figure 9–1). The term *ventricular premature beat (VPB)* means the same thing.

Premature ventricular beats are often followed by a compensatory pause, since the next atrial beat may not be conducted through refractory junctional tissue.

54 ◻ SECTION I: SYSTEMATIC APPROACH TO ECGs

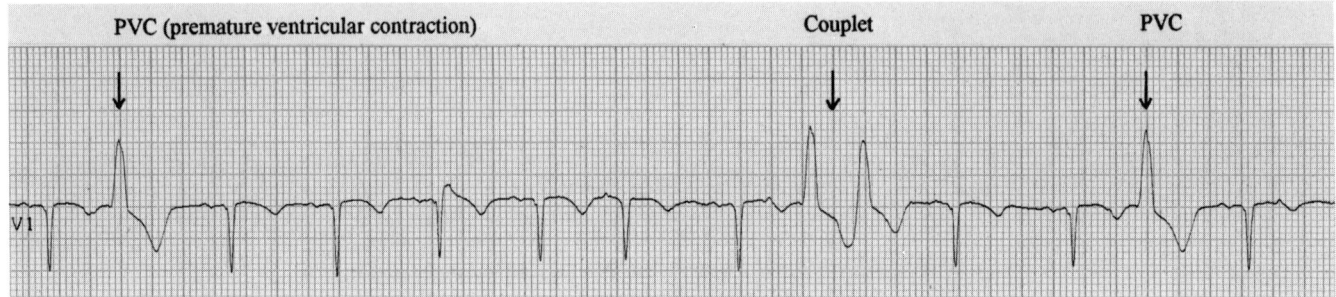

FIGURE 9–1. Ventricular ectopic activity

If every other beat is a PVC, there is *bigeminy;* if every third beat is a PVC, there is *trigeminy;* and so on (Figure 9–2).

If the PVCs originate from the same ectopic focus, they are *unifocal,* whereas PVCs of different morphologies are *multifocal.*

B. Ventricular Tachycardia

Couplets are two PVCs in immediate succession (see Figure 9–1); more than this are *salvos* or *runs.* If the entire rhythm consists of ventricular beats at a rate over 120 beats per minute, the rhythm is *ventricular tachycardia (VT).* If VT occurs for more than 30 seconds, it is termed *sustained VT,* whereas if it terminates in less than 30 seconds, it is *nonsustained VT.* VT may degenerate into ventricular fibrillation.

VT occurs in ischemic heart disease and severe left ventricular dysfunction, but it also can happen in the absence of structural heart disease. The mechanism of VT may be reentry within the ventricles or automaticity of a ventricular focus.

In VT, P waves are unrelated to QRS complexes, and there is AV dissociation. VT may be difficult to distinguish from supraventricular tachycardia with aberrancy.

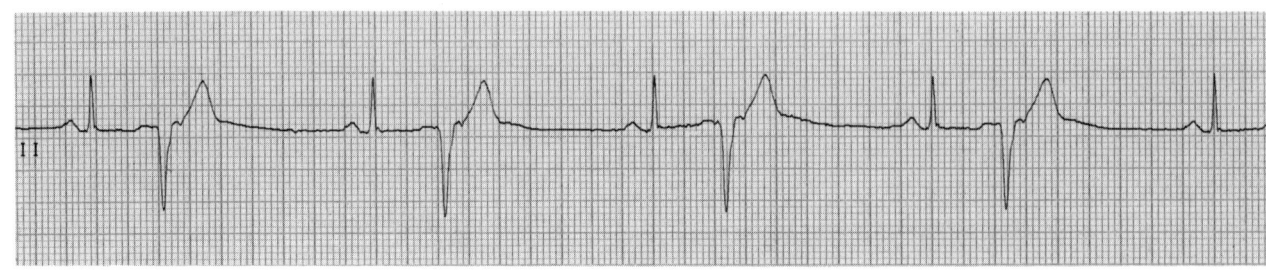

FIGURE 9–2. Ventricular bigeminy

C. Idioventricular Rhythm (Figure 9–3)

If electrical impulses from the pacemaker centers in the SA node or the junctional tissues do not reach the ventricles, pacemaker centers in the ventricular tissue will fire at their intrinsic rate of 30 to 40 beats per minute. This is called an *idioventricular rhythm*.

If a ventricular rhythm occurs faster than 30 to 40 beats per minute but slower than 120 beats per minute, it is an *accelerated idioventricular rhythm (AIVR)*. AIVR is not as worrisome as ventricular tachycardia.

D. Ventricular Fibrillation

Ventricular fibrillation (VF) occurs when the ventricles fibrillate chaotically, with no effective ventricular contraction. The ECG shows an undulating baseline with no recognizable QRS complexes. VF is a preterminal event if left untreated.

E. Torsades de Pointes

Torsades de pointes, literally "twisting of the points," is a rapid, somewhat irregular VT where the axis of the QRS complex varies. It occurs in association with a prolonged QT interval. It has been associated with medications that prolong the QT interval such as quinidine and tricyclic antidepressants, as well as with hypomagnesemia.

True torsades occurs only in the setting of a prolonged QT interval (more than 0.5s). Otherwise, a varying axis in VT is probably *polymorphous VT*, which does not behave as torsades.

Torsades de pointes may degenerate into VF and is very refractory to conventional antiarrhythmics.

III. ABERRANCY

A. The Concept of Aberrancy

Wide QRS complexes may be ventricular in origin or supraventricular with aberrant conduction.

Aberrantly conducted beats occur when the myocardium has not yet fully repolarized from the last contraction.

The right bundle is often more refractory than the left bundle, so the most common appearance of aberrantly conducted beats is in RBBB. The initial deflection of the QRS is most commonly the same as that of a normal beat.

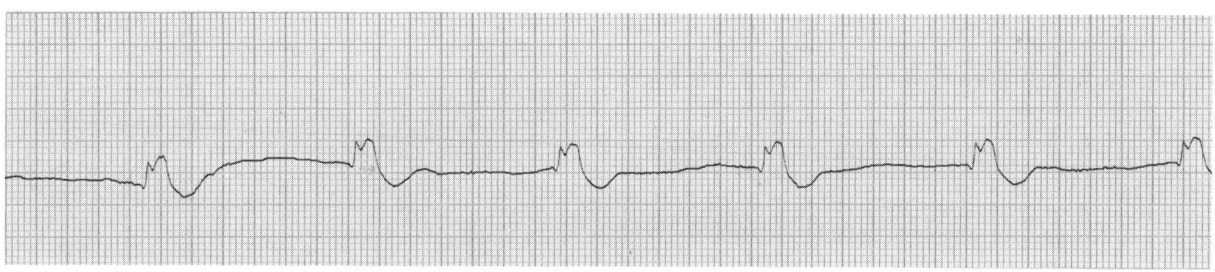

Figure 9–3. Idioventricular rhythm

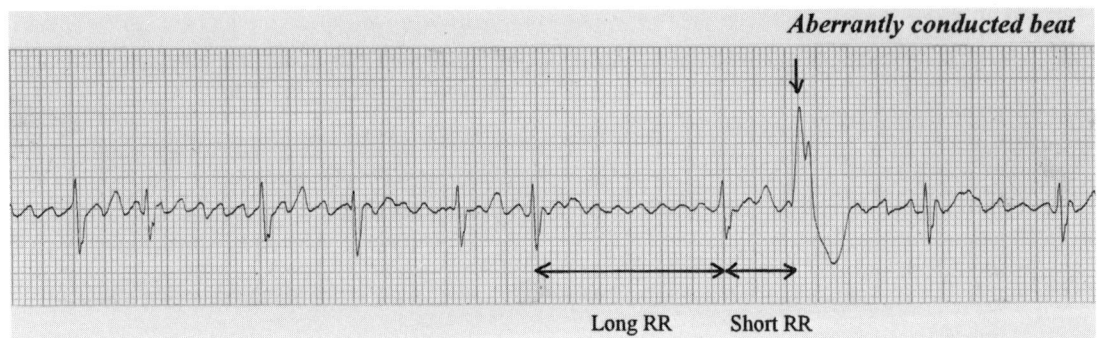

Figure 9–4. Aberrant conduction in coarse atrial fibrillation

B. Ashman Beats

Ashman beats are aberrantly conducted QRS complexes in atrial fibrillation following a "long–short" cycle (Figure 9–4).

The QT interval represents ventricular repolarization and is determined by the *preceding* R-R interval. After a long R-R interval, the ventricle may still be refractory, and an early supraventricular impulse (short R-R) may lead to aberrancy.

How can you tell if a wide complex is actually a PVC rather than aberrantly conducted? If there is a wide beat following a long–short cycle, look for an R-R interval elsewhere on the tracing that is at least as long, followed by an R-R that is at least as short. If the QRS after the short interval is normal, then the ventricle *can* conduct normally, so the wide beat must be ventricular.

C. Ventricular Tachycardia versus Aberrant SVT

It may be very difficult to distinguish between ventricular tachycardia and supraventricular tachycardia with aberrancy. Although there are numerous articles in the literature about findings that favor one diagnosis over the other, they are not absolutely accurate.

It can never be *proven* that a wide QRS is aberrant, but it may be possible to find evidence that a wide QRS is ventricular in origin. Generally, the finding of AV dissociation, either electrocardiographically or by physical examination, proves that the wide complexes are ventricular.

IV. SUMMARY

Wide QRS complexes arise either from the ventricles or from a supraventricular source with aberrant conduction.

In atrial fibrillation, aberrant conduction occurs when the ventricles are refractory after a long R-R interval and receive an early impulse, a short R-R interval.

It may be difficult to distinguish between ventricular tachycardia and supraventricular tachycardia with aberrancy. Evidence of AV dissociation is the best evidence that a wide QRS is ventricular in origin.

Chapter 10

DRUGS AND METABOLIC DISORDERS

I. INTRODUCTION

This chapter presents the electrocardiographic effects of certain drugs, electrolyte abnormalities, and pericardial processes.

After completing this chapter, you should be able to

1. Recognize the effects of digoxin, quinidine, and phenothiazines.
2. Recognize the electrocardiographic findings of hypokalemia, hyperkalemia, hypocalcemia, and hypercalcemia.
3. Recognize the findings associated with pericarditis and pericardial effusion.

II. DRUGS

A. Digitalis

Digitalis is given to cardiac patients for two major reasons:

1. To slow conduction through the AV node.
2. To increase myocardial contractility in heart failure.

Slowing of AV nodal conduction is useful in atrial fibrillation, where it brings the ventricular response down to a reasonable rate, and in supraventricular tachyarrhythmias that involve conduction through the AV node, such as PSVT, where it may interrupt the arrhythmia.

The normal effect of digoxin is sagging or scooping ST-segment depression (see Figure 10–1). A prolonged PR interval also can be seen.

The effects of toxic levels of digoxin are many and include
  Sinus bradycardia
  AV block (first, second, or third degree)
  Atrial fibrillation with slow ventricular response
  Accelerated junctional tachycardia
  PAT, often with AV block
  Ventricular ectopy, VT, VF

Patients in atrial fibrillation who develop accelerated junctional tachycardia go from an irregular rhythm (AF) to a regular rhythm (junctional tachycardia); because they still have no P waves, they are often said to have *regularization of ventricular response*. This arrhythmia should immediately raise the suspicion of digoxin toxicity, although other causes that irritate the junctional tissues may lead to the same rhythm.

B. Quinidine

Normal quinidine effects include QRS prolongation, ST-segment depression, T-wave inversion, and QT prolongation.

Toxic rhythms include ventricular ectopy and polymorphous VT, which in the setting of a prolonged QT interval is torsades de pointes.

C. Tricyclic Antidepressants and Phenothiazines

Tricyclic antidepressants and phenothiazines have similar effects as quinidine. They prolong the QRS duration and the QT interval and cause ST-segment depression and T-wave inversion. In overdoses of tricyclic antidepressants, the *QRS duration* is more prognostically important than the absolute level of the drug. The QRS duration acts as a bioassay of the effects of the drug. See Figure 10–2 for an example of QT prolongation.

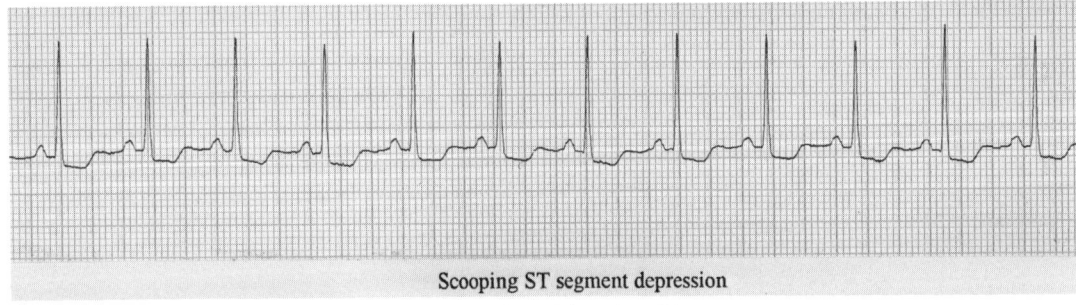

Scooping ST segment depression

FIGURE 10–1. Digoxin effect

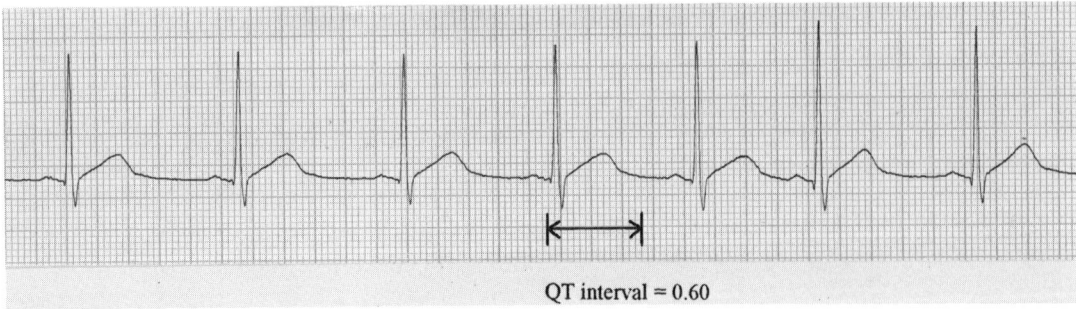

QT interval = 0.60

FIGURE 10–2. QT prolongation, typical of quinidine effect

III. ELECTROLYTE ABNORMALITIES

A. Hyperkalemia (Figure 10–3)

Increasing serum concentrations of potassium lead to the following changes:
 Tall, peaked T waves
 AV conduction problems and flat P waves that may be difficult to see
 Prolonged QRS complex duration
 ST-segment depression and T-wave inversion
 VT and VF

B. Hypokalemia (Figure 10–4)

Hypokalemia leads to ST-segment depression and T-wave flattening. With serum potassium levels less than 3.0, prominent U waves will be seen. These are due to continued ventricular repolarization, but they follow the T wave.

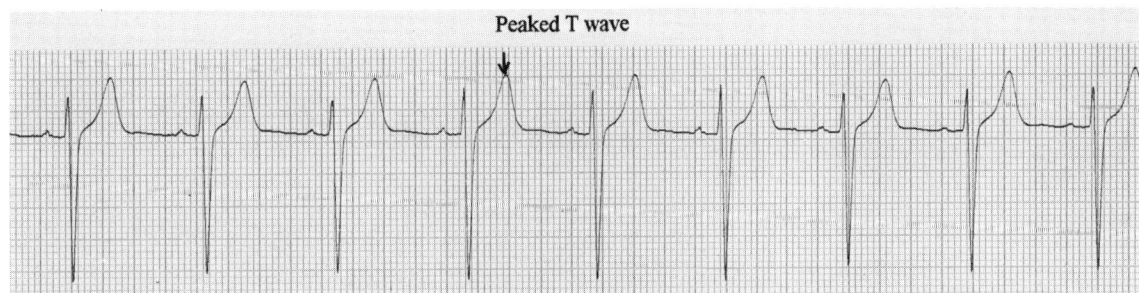

FIGURE 10–3. Hyperkalemia: Peaked T waves

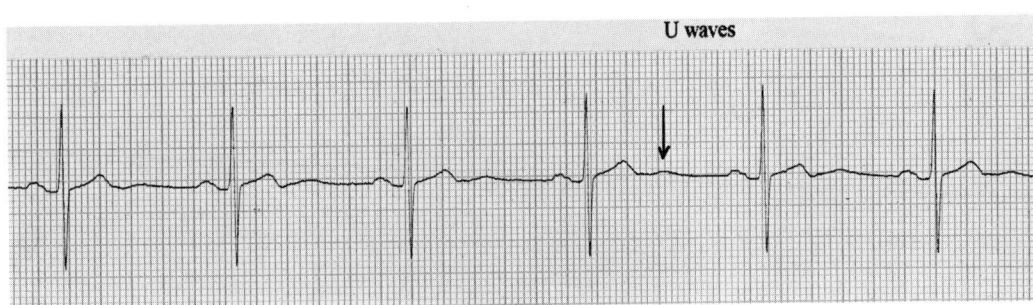

FIGURE 10–4. Hypokalemia: U waves

60 □ SECTION I: SYSTEMATIC APPROACH TO ECGs

C. Hypercalcemia (Figure 10–5)

Hypercalcemia leads to a shortened QT interval, with the T wave arising abruptly from the QRS.

D. Hypocalcemia (Figure 10–6)

Hypocalcemia leads to a prolonged QT interval. However, in contrast to the effects of quinidine, the T-wave duration remains normal and the ST segment is prolonged. If the hypocalcemia is severe, there may be T-wave inversion as well.

IV. PERICARDIAL PROCESSES

A. Pericarditis (Figure 10–7)

Pericarditis is an inflammation of the pericardium. The changes seen on ECG are ST-segment elevation and PR-interval depression. The baseline of the tracing should be taken as the segment

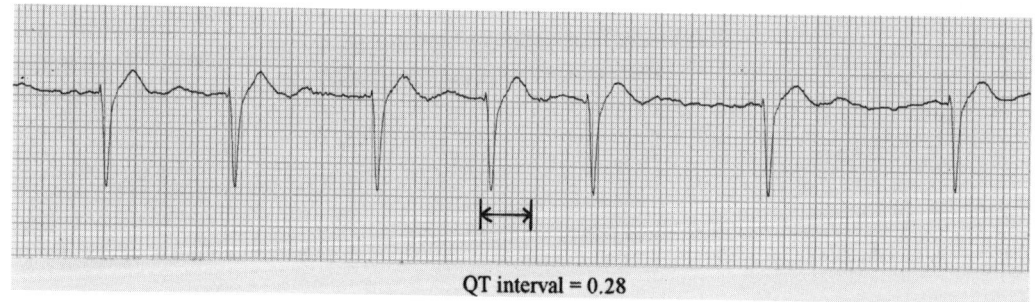

FIGURE 10–5. Hypercalcemia: Short QT interval with sharp upstroke

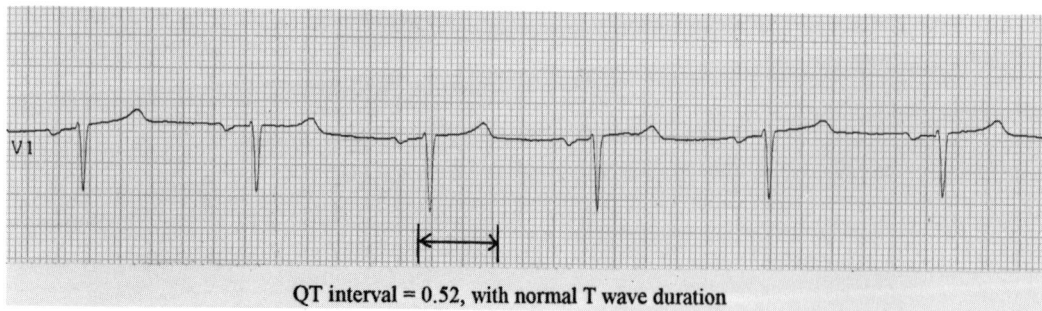

FIGURE 10–6. Hypocalcemia: Prolonged QT interval with normal T wave duration

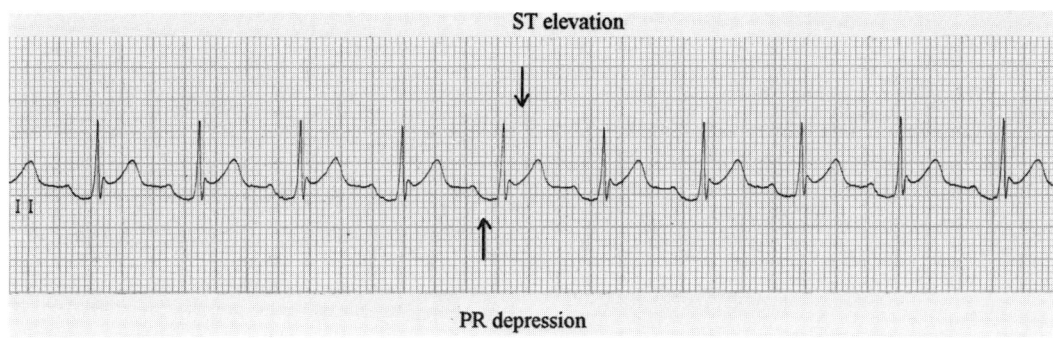

Figure 10–7. Pericarditis

between one T wave and the next P wave. If the PR segment is below this level, there is PR-interval depression.

B. Pericardial Effusion

Pericardial effusions may cause low voltage because of the fluid that comes between the heart and the electrodes on the chest. There also may be *electrical alternans,* in which the size of the QRS complex varies from beat to beat.

V. SUMMARY

Drugs and electrolyte abnormalities may have the typical electrocardiographic features listed in this chapter. However, these features are not pathognomonic, and the interpretation of any changes should be carried out in the context of the clinical history.

SECTION II

Practice ECG Tracings

CASE 1

Rate and Rhythm

There is a P wave preceding each QRS complex, and the rhythm is normal sinus rhythm.

The heart rate is about 90 beats per minute (bpm).

Intervals

PR interval: 0.16s
QRS duration: 0.08s
QT interval: 0.36s

QRS Axis

The QRS complex is positive in lead I and negative in lead aVF. The QRS axis is therefore in the leftward quadrant. The isoelectric lead is II, so the QRS axis is about −30 degrees. This is left axis deviation.

Evidence for Atrial Enlargement

In lead II, the P wave is wider than 2.5 mm and is notched. In lead V1, the P wave is biphasic, with the terminal component wider than 1 mm. Thus there are criteria for left atrial enlargement in both leads II and V1.

Evidence for Ventricular Hypertrophy

LVH: The sum of the S wave in V1 (8 mm) and the R wave in V6 (7 mm) is 15 mm. There is no evidence for left ventricular hypertrophy by voltage criteria.

RVH: The QRS axis is in the leftward quadrant. There is no evidence for right ventricular hypertrophy.

R-Wave Progression

R waves are present in V1 through V6, but they do not grow very much from V1 to V5. The QRS complex does not become mostly positive until V6. Therefore, there is poor R-wave progression. In this tracing, the likely causes are anteroseptal MI, clockwise rotation, and faulty lead placement.

Evidence of Ischemia or Infarction

Anterior leads: There is poor R-wave progression, which may indicate an old anteroseptal MI. There are no acute ST-segment elevations, which would suggest that the MI is acute, nor are there ST-segment depressions or T-wave inversions, which would indicate ischemia.

Inferior leads: There are Q waves in leads II, III, and aVF consistent with an inferior MI. There is no ST-segment elevation, so there is no evidence that it is acute.

Summary

Normal sinus rhythm at 90 bpm
Intervals: 0.16/0.08/0.36
Axis: −30 degrees
Left axis deviation
Left atrial enlargement
Poor R-wave progression consistent with old anteroseptal MI, clockwise rotation, or faulty lead placement
Q waves in leads II, III, and aVF consistent with old inferior MI

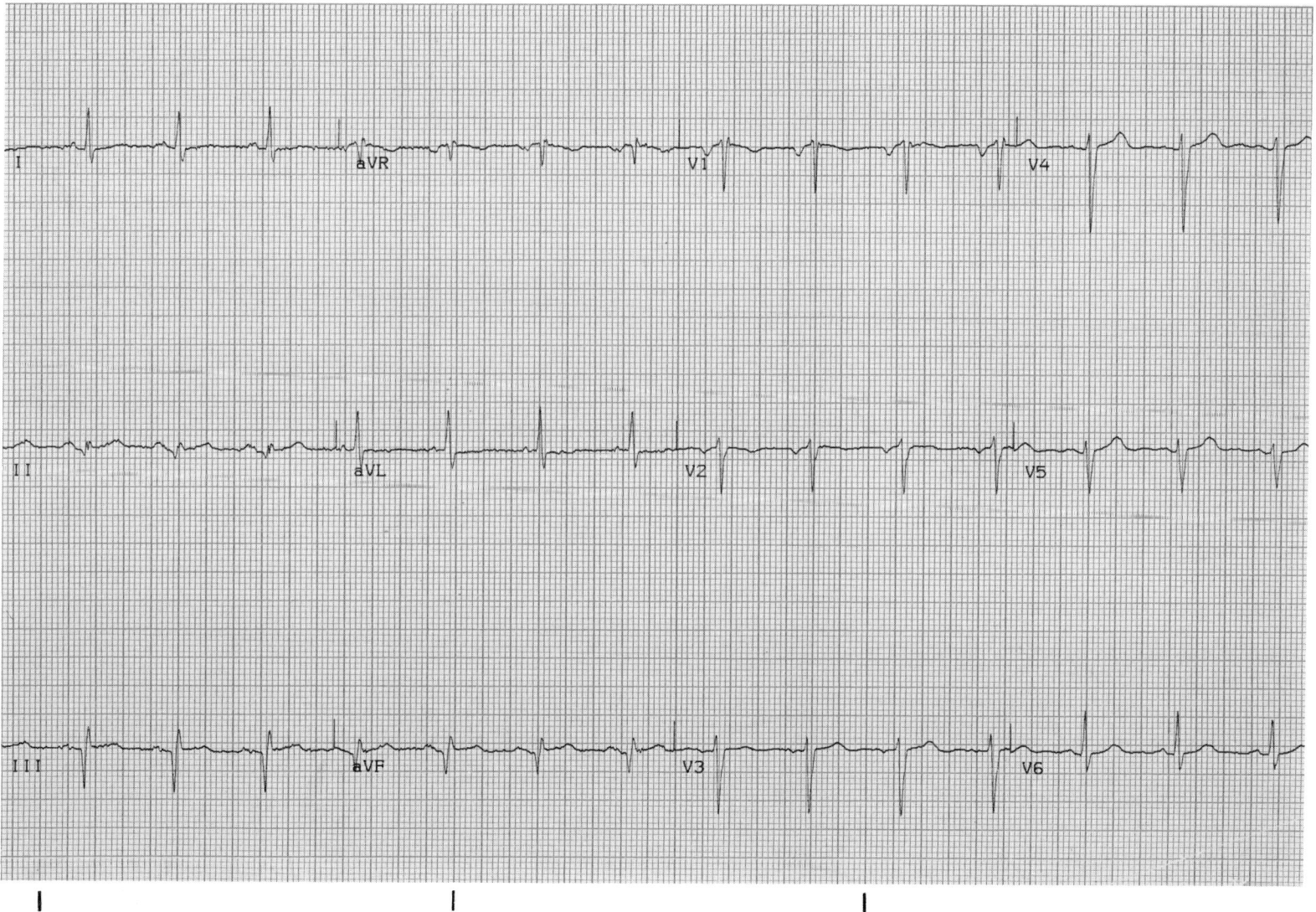

CASE 2

Rate and Rhythm

There is a P wave preceding each QRS complex, and the rhythm is normal sinus rhythm.

The heart rate is about 100 beats per minute.

Intervals

PR interval: 0.16s
QRS duration: 0.08s
QT interval: 0.32s

QRS Axis

The QRS complex is positive in lead I and positive in lead aVF, so the QRS axis is in the normal quadrant. Leads III and aVL are the closest to isoelectric. If lead III were isoelectric, the QRS axis would be +30 degrees, and if lead aVL were isoelectric, the axis would be +60 degrees. The QRS axis is between the two, about +45 degrees.

Evidence for Atrial Enlargement

There is no evidence for atrial enlargement.

Evidence for Ventricular Hypertrophy

LVH: The sum of the S wave in V1 (12 mm) and the R wave in V5 (13 mm) is 25 mm. There is no evidence of left ventricular hypertrophy by voltage criteria.

RVH: The QRS axis is in the normal quadrant. There is no evidence for right ventricular hypertrophy.

R-Wave Progression

The R waves grow in size from V1 to V4. The transition point at which the QRS becomes mostly positive is between V3 and V4, so there is good (normal) R-wave progression.

Evidence of Ischemia or Infarction

Anterior leads: There is no evidence of ischemia or infarction.
Inferior leads: There is no evidence of ischemia or infarction.
ST-T waves: The T waves in both anterior and inferior leads are not entirely normal, but the abnormalities are not specific for ischemia and they do not appear to be secondary changes of hypertrophy or bundle-branch block. Thus there are nonspecific ST-T wave abnormalities.

Summary

Normal sinus rhythm at 100 bpm
Intervals: 0.16/0.08/0.32
QRS axis: +45 degrees
Nonspecific ST-T wave abnormalities

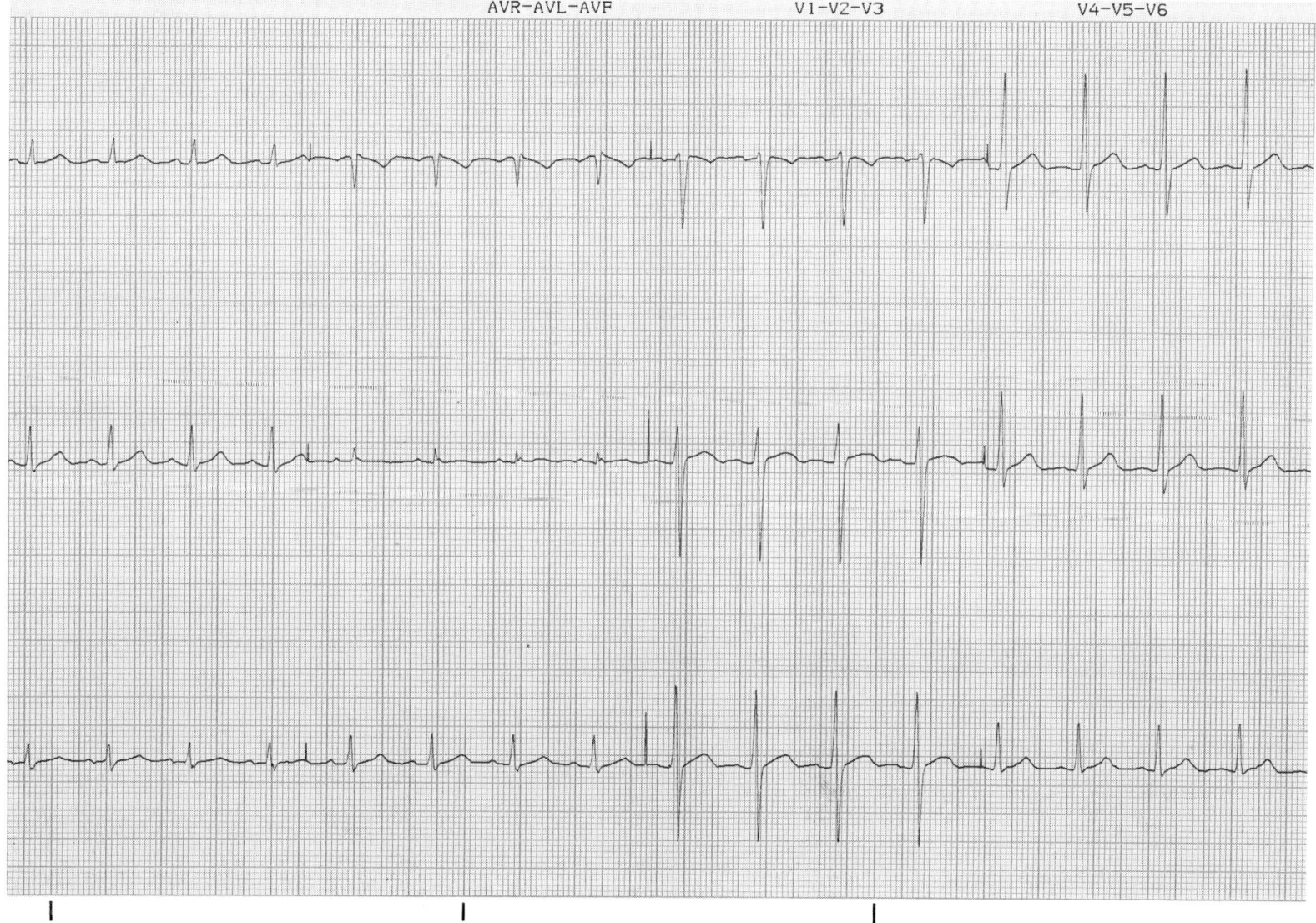

CASE 3

Rate and Rhythm

There is a P wave preceding each QRS complex, and the rhythm is normal sinus rhythm.

The heart rate is about 90 beats per minute.

Intervals

PR interval: 0.16s
QRS duration: 0.08s
QT interval: 0.36s

QRS Axis

The QRS complex is positive in lead I and positive in lead aVF, so the QRS axis is in the normal quadrant. The isoelectric lead is III, so the QRS axis is +30 degrees.

Evidence for Atrial Enlargement

The P waves are difficult to see in lead II. In lead V1, the P wave is biphasic and the first part of the P wave is almost 1 mm wide, which is a criterion for right atrial enlargement. However, lead II does not show peaked P waves greater than 2.5 mm in height that are typical of right atrial enlargement. Thus we would not specifically comment on atrial enlargement.

Evidence for Ventricular Hypertrophy

LVH: The sum of the S wave in V1 (9 mm) and the R wave in V5 (22 mm) is 31 mm. There is no evidence of left ventricular hypertrophy by voltage criteria.

RVH: The QRS axis is in the normal quadrant. There is no evidence for right ventricular hypertrophy.

R-Wave Progression

The R waves grow in size from V1 to V5. The transition point at which the QRS becomes mostly positive occurs at V3. Thus there is good R-wave progression.

Evidence of Ischemia or Infarction

Anterior leads: There is good R-wave progression and there are no changes that suggest ischemia or infarction. There are small *q* waves in V5 and V6 that are septal *q* waves.

Inferior leads: There is T-wave inversion in lead III alone. The T waves in leads II and aVF are flattened, but there is no specific evidence of ischemia or infarction.

ST-T waves: The ST segments in leads V5 and V6 suggest normal early repolarization. The inferior T-wave changes, if we were to specifically comment on them, would be nonspecific ST-T wave abnormalities.

Summary

Normal sinus rhythm at 90 bpm
Intervals: 0.16/0.08/0.36
QRS axis: +30 degrees
Tracing is within normal limits
Normal early repolarization and nonspecific ST-T wave abnormalities (optional)

CASE 3 □ 69

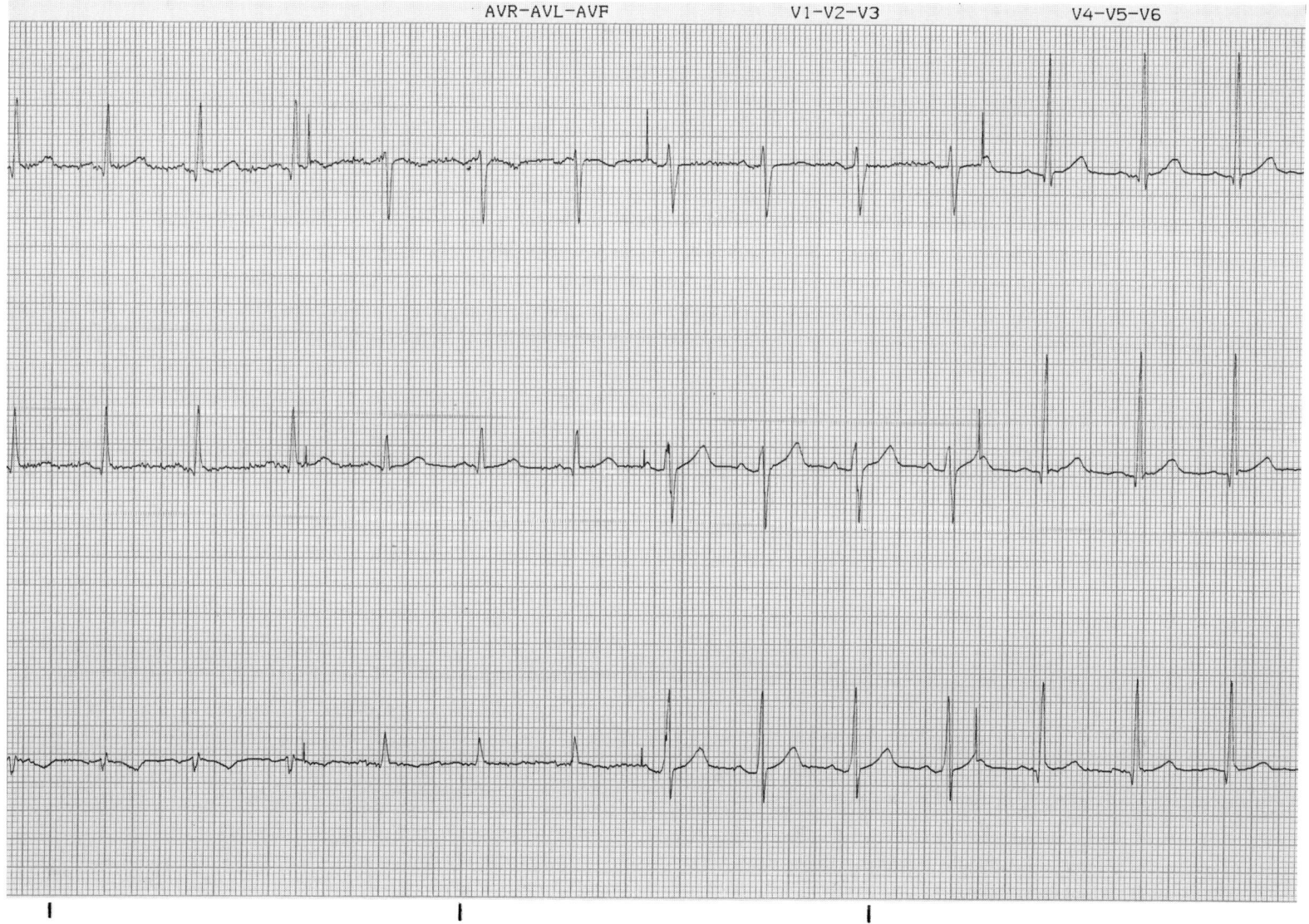

CASE 4

Rate and Rhythm

There is a P wave preceding each QRS complex, and the rhythm is normal sinus rhythm.

The heart rate is about 75 beats per minute.

Intervals

PR interval: 0.20s
QRS duration: 0.06s
QT interval: 0.36s

QRS Axis

The QRS complex is positive in lead I and negative in lead aVF, so the QRS axis is in the leftward quadrant. Leads II and aVF are closest to isoelectric, so the QRS axis is between 0 and −30 degrees, or about −15 degrees. This is "leftward axis" but is *not* left axis deviation.

Evidence for Atrial Enlargement

The P waves appear broad in lead II but do not show changes typical of left atrial enlargement in lead V1. Thus we will make no specific comment about atrial enlargement.

Evidence for Ventricular Hypertrophy

LVH: The sum of the S wave in V1 (8 mm) and the R wave in V5 (21 mm) is 29 mm. There is no evidence of left ventricular hypertrophy by voltage criteria.

RVH: The QRS axis is in the leftward quadrant. There is no evidence for right ventricular hypertrophy.

R-Wave Progression

The R waves grow in size from V1 to V5. The transition point occurs at V4, so there is good R-wave progression.

Evidence of Ischemia or Infarction

Anterior leads: There is good R-wave progression in the anterior leads. However, there are downsloping ST-segment depressions in V1, V2, and V3 that are consistent with anterior ischemia or subendocardial infarction. There are also downsloping ST-segment depressions in leads V6, I, and aV$_L$ consistent with apicolateral ischemia or subendocardial infarction.

Inferior leads: There is marked ST-segment elevation in leads II, III, and aVF suggesting an acute inferior MI. There are Q waves in aVF already. Given the evidence of inferior injury, the anterior ST-segment depressions seen in V1 to V3 also may reflect reciprocal changes of posterior injury as well.

Summary

Normal sinus rhythm at 75 bpm
Intervals: 0.20/0.06/0.36
QRS axis: −15 degrees
ST-segment elevation in leads II, III, and aVF suggesting acute inferior MI
ST-segment depression in leads V6, I, and aVL suggesting apicolateral ischemia or subendocardial infarction
ST-segment depression in leads V1 to V3 consistent with either anterior ischemia or posterior injury

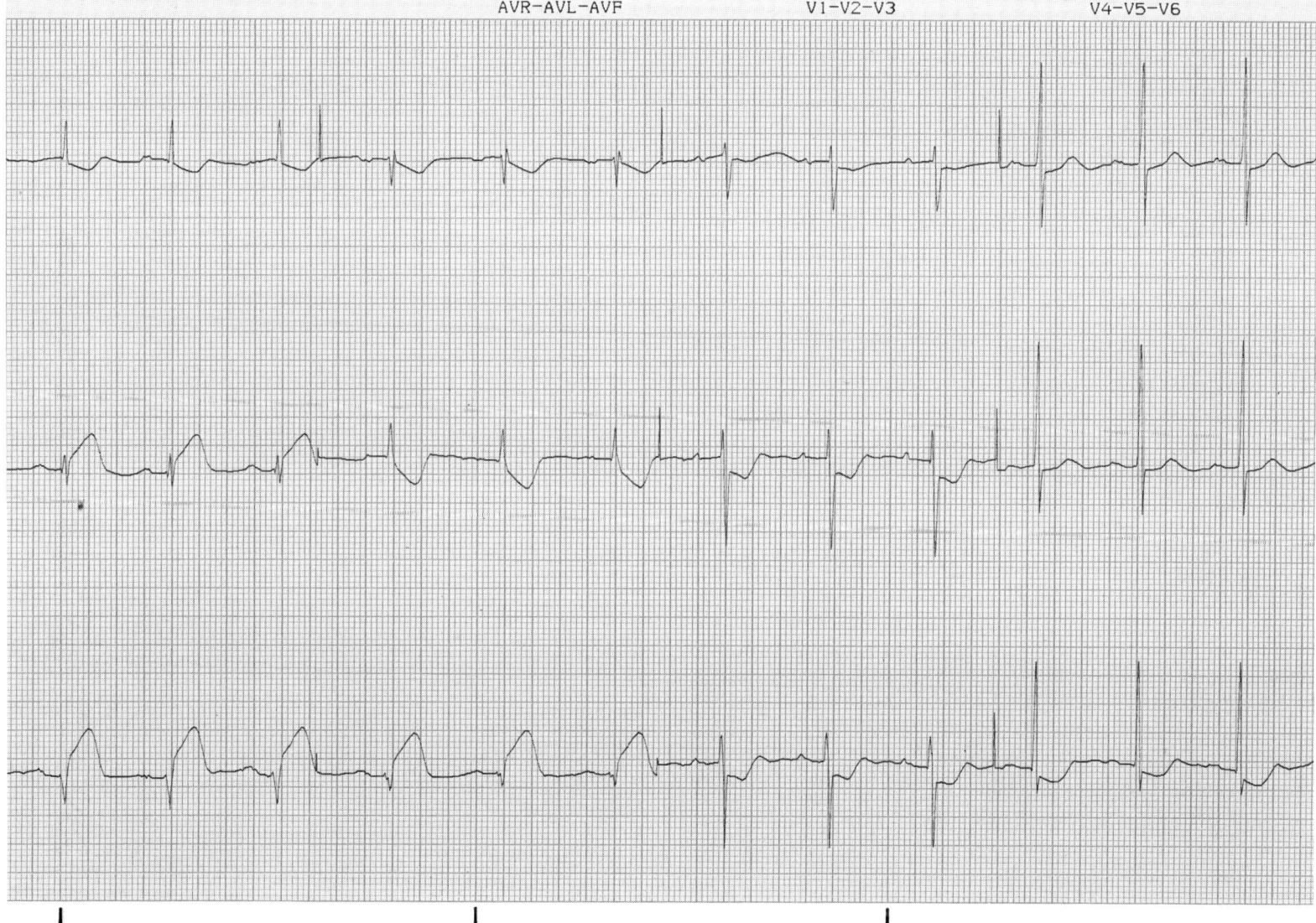

CASE 5

Rate and Rhythm

There is a P wave preceding each QRS complex, and the rhythm is normal sinus rhythm.

The heart rate is 65 to 70 beats per minute.

Intervals

PR interval: 0.16s
QRS duration: 0.12s
QT interval: 0.40s

The prolonged QRS duration tells us that there is a bundle-branch block. Looking at V1, we see that there is an RSR' pattern typical of right bundle-branch block.

QRS Axis

The QRS complex is positive in lead I and negative in lead aVF, so the QRS axis is in the leftward quadrant. Leads II and aVR are closest to isoelectric. If lead II were isoelectric, the QRS axis would be −30 degrees. If lead aVR were isoelectric, the QRS axis would be −60 degrees. The QRS axis is between the two, or about −45 degrees. This is left axis deviation. In the absence of left bundle-branch block and left ventricular hypertrophy, the left axis deviation suggests left anterior hemiblock.

Evidence for Atrial Enlargement

The P wave in lead II is notched and widened to 2.5 mm. The P wave in lead V1 is biphasic, with the latter part about 1 mm in width. Thus, in both leads II and V1, there is evidence for borderline left atrial enlargement.

Evidence for Ventricular Hypertrophy

In the presence of right bundle-branch block, we cannot assess criteria for ventricular hypertrophy.

R-Wave Progression

In the presence of right bundle-branch block, we can assess R-wave progression if we look at only the first part of the QRS complexes (the R waves, not the R' waves). The R waves grow in size from V1 to V6. Although we cannot assess the transition point accurately because of the bundle-branch block, there does not appear to be evidence for poor R-wave progression.

Evidence of Ischemia or Infarction

Anterior leads: There is no specific evidence for ischemia or infarction.
Inferior leads: There is T-wave inversion in leads II, III, and aVF consistent with inferior ischemia or subendocardial infarction. These are not due to the right bundle-branch block alone.
ST-T waves: There are secondary changes from the right bundle-branch block.

Summary

Normal sinus rhythm at 65 to 70 bpm
Intervals: 0.16/0.12/0.40
QRS axis: −45 degrees
Borderline left atrial enlargement
Right bundle-branch block and left anterior hemiblock
T-wave inversion in leads II, III, and aVF consistent with inferior ischemia or subendocardial infarction

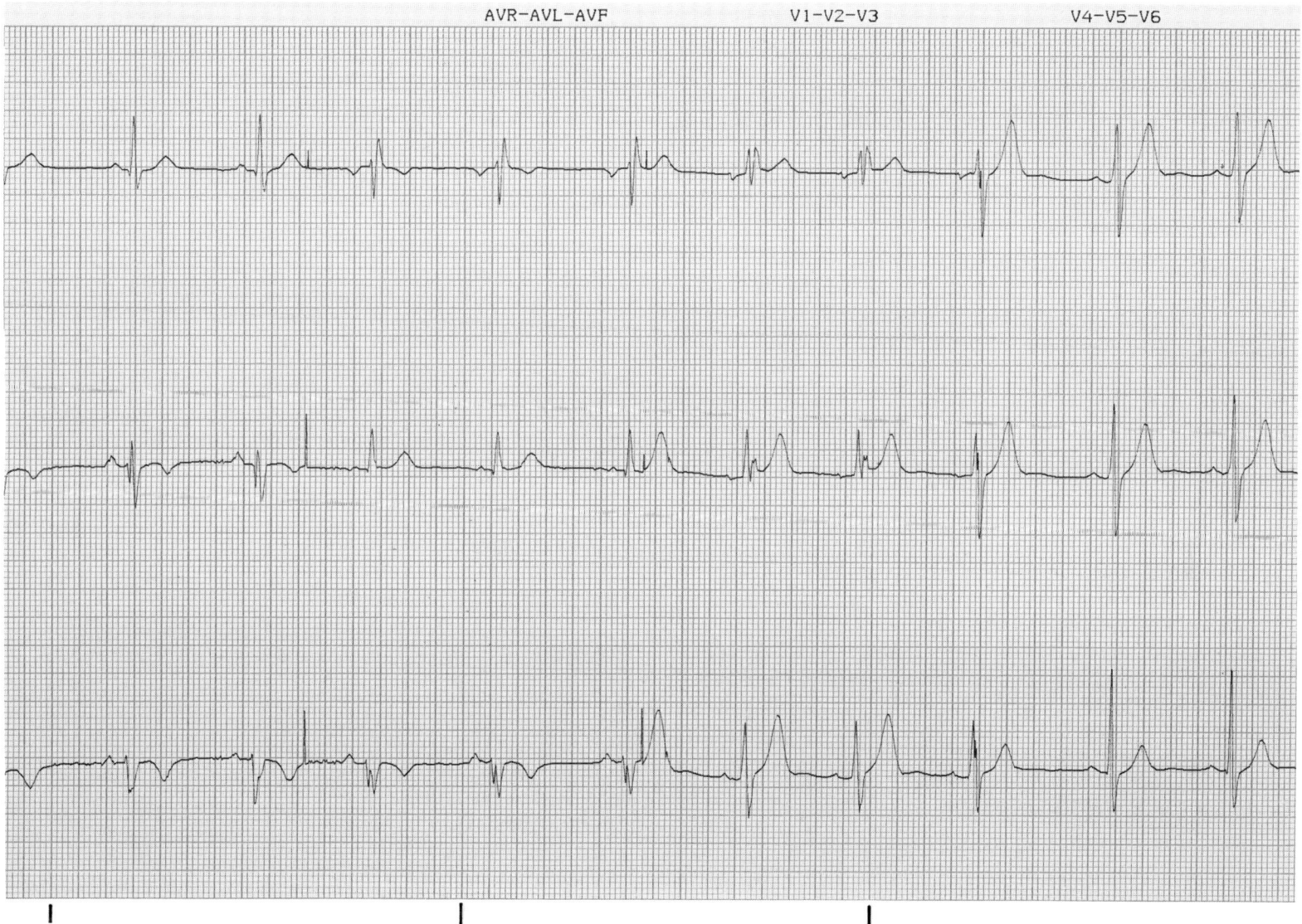

CASE 6

Rate and Rhythm

There is a P wave preceding each QRS complex, and the rhythm is normal sinus rhythm.

The heart rate is about 70 beats per minute.

Intervals

PR interval: 0.12s
QRS duration: 0.12s
QT interval: 0.36s

The prolonged QRS duration tells us that there is a bundle-branch block. Looking at V1, we see that there is an RSR' pattern typical of right bundle-branch block.

QRS Axis

The QRS complex is positive in lead I and negative in lead aVF, so the QRS axis is in the leftward quadrant. Leads II and aVR are the closest to isoelectric, so the QRS axis is between −30 and −60 degrees, or about −45 degrees. This is left axis deviation. In the absence of left ventricular hypertrophy and left bundle-branch block, left axis deviation is consistent with left anterior hemiblock.

Evidence for Atrial Enlargement

The P wave in lead II is 2 mm wide, and the P wave in V1 is biphasic, with the terminal portion about 1 mm wide. These findings suggest left atrial enlargement but do not meet the criteria.

Evidence for Ventricular Hypertrophy

In the presence of right bundle-branch block, we cannot assess criteria for ventricular hypertrophy.

R-Wave Progression

Looking only at the first part of the QRS complexes, we see that there is a very small R wave in V1 and a frank Q wave in V2. Thus there is poor R-wave progression, and the findings suggest an anteroseptal MI.

Evidence of Ischemia or Infarction

Anterior leads: There is poor R-wave progression with a Q wave in V2, suggesting an anteroseptal MI. The T waves in V2 are biphasic, and there is T-wave inversion in V3 to V6, suggesting anterior ischemia or subendocardial infarction. The ST segments in V6, I, and aVL are flat to slightly inverted as well. These changes are not due to right bundle-branch block alone.

Inferior leads: The T waves are flat in II, III, and aVF, suggesting possible inferior ischemia.

Summary

Normal sinus rhythm at 70 bpm
Intervals: 0.12/0.12/0.36
QRS axis: −45 degrees
Right bundle-branch block and left anterior hemiblock
Poor R-wave progression with a Q wave in V2 consistent with anteroseptal MI
T-wave inversion in V3 to V5 consistent with anterior ischemia or subendocardial infarction
T-wave flattening in II, III, and aVF, as well as in V6, I, and aVL, consistent with inferior and apicolateral ischemia

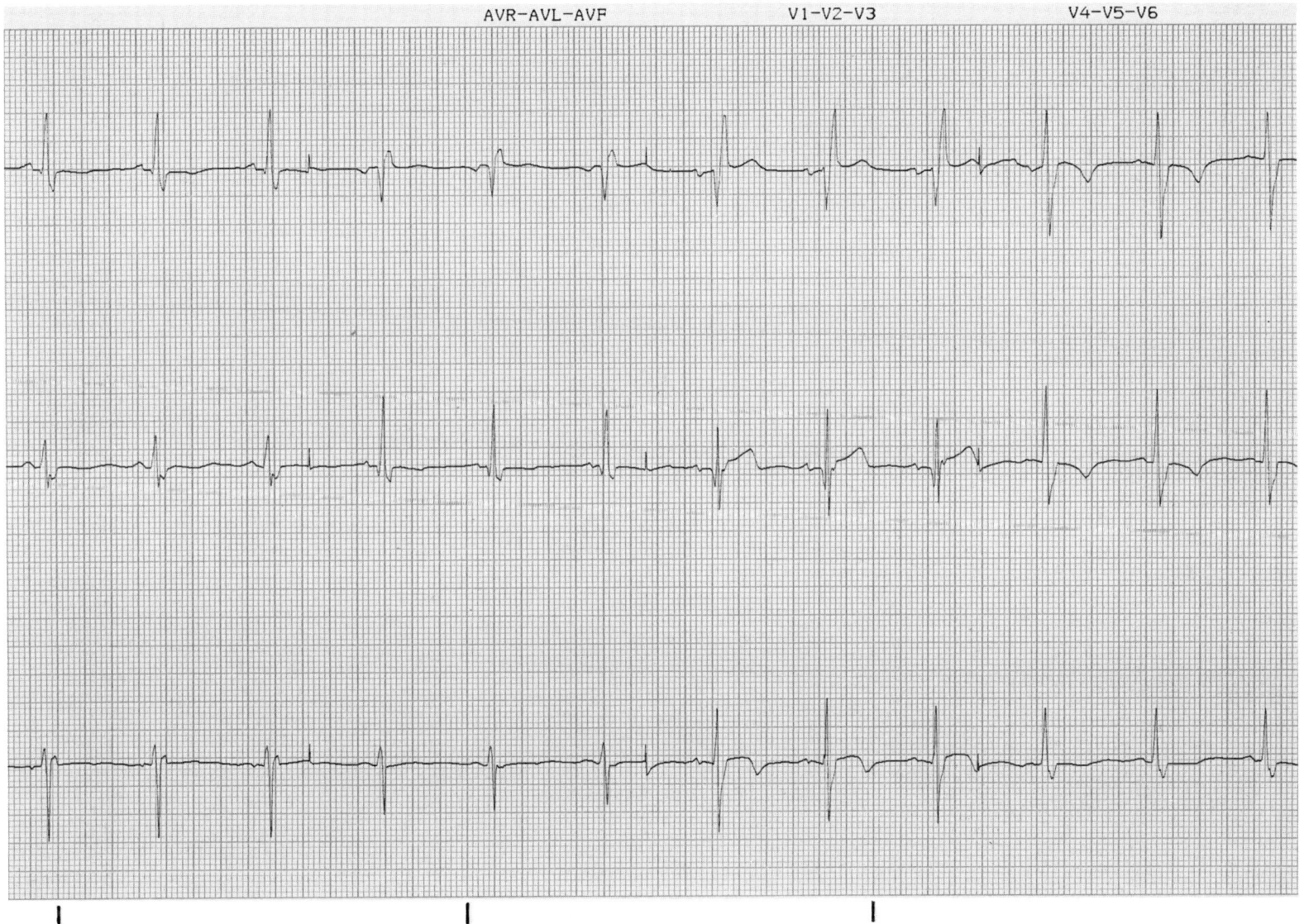

CASE 7

Rate and Rhythm

There is a P wave preceding each QRS complex, and the rhythm is normal sinus rhythm. There are two wide QRS complexes, which are premature ventricular beats. Notice how the sinus rhythm is uninterrupted by the premature ventricular beats.

The heart rate of the sinus rhythm is about 60 beats per minute.

Intervals

PR interval: 0.16s
QRS duration: 0.10s
QT interval: 0.36s

The QRS duration is at the upper limit of normal, so we may say that there is an interventricular conduction delay.

QRS Axis

The QRS complex is positive in lead I and negative in lead aVF, so the QRS axis is in the leftward axis quadrant. The isoelectric lead is II, so the QRS axis is −30 degrees. This is left axis deviation, consistent with left anterior hemiblock.

Evidence for Atrial Enlargement

In lead II, the P wave is wide, measuring about 2.5 mm. In lead V1, the P wave is biphasic, and the terminal negative part is 1 mm wide. Thus there is evidence in both leads II and V1 for left atrial enlargement.

Evidence for Ventricular Hypertrophy

LVH: The sum of the S wave in V1 (5 mm) and the R wave in V5 (17 mm) is 22 mm. There is no evidence of left ventricular hypertrophy by voltage criteria.

RVH: The QRS axis is in the normal quadrant. There is no evidence for right ventricular hypertrophy.

R-Wave Progression

The R waves grow from V1 to V5 and become mostly positive in V4. Thus there is normal R-wave progression.

Evidence of Ischemia or Infarction

Anterior leads: There is no evidence for ischemia or infarction in the anterior leads.

Inferior leads: There is an isolated inverted T wave in lead III, which is a normal variant. The T waves in II and aVF are normal. Thus there is no evidence for ischemia or infarction in the inferior leads.

Summary

Normal sinus rhythm at 60 bpm, with occasional premature ventricular beats
Intervals: 0.16/0.10/0.36
QRS axis: −30 degrees
Left axis deviation consistent with left anterior hemiblock
Interventricular conduction delay (optional)

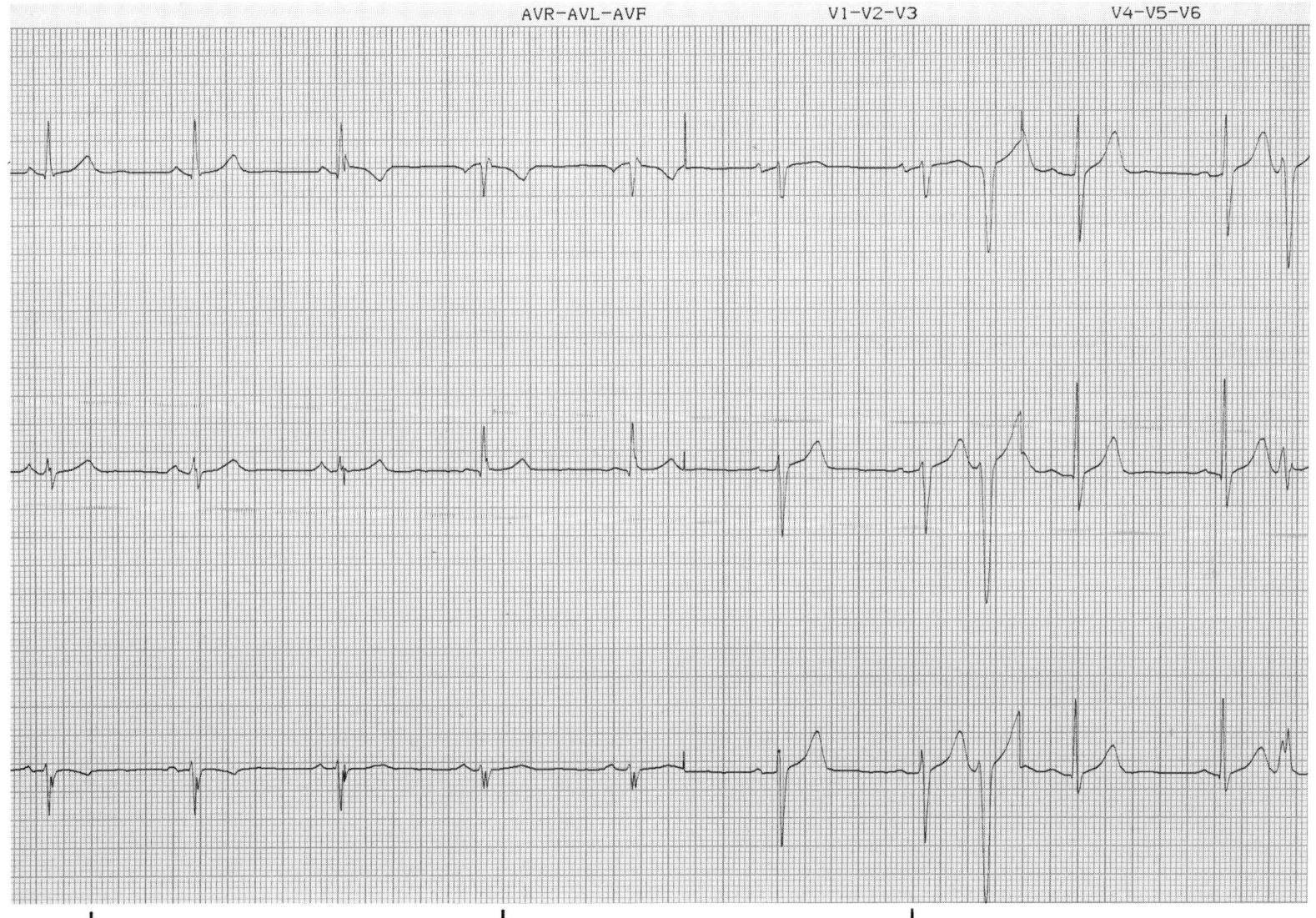

CASE 8

Rate and Rhythm

There is a P wave preceding each QRS complex, so the rhythm is sinus rhythm.

The heart rate is about 50 beats per minute. There is a pause in the rhythm between the fourth and fifth QRS complexes. Following the pattern of the first four complexes, the next one is missing, but the one following that comes in right on time. This is sinus exit block.

Intervals

PR interval: 0.28s
QRS duration: 0.08s
QT interval: 0.44s

The prolonged PR interval tells us that there is first-degree AV block. Because there are no P waves that are not followed by QRS complexes, there is no second-degree AV block.

QRS Axis

The QRS complex is positive in lead I and positive in lead aVF, so the QRS axis is in the normal quadrant. The isoelectric lead is between III and aVF, so the QRS axis is about +15 degrees.

Evidence for Atrial Enlargement

In lead II, the P wave is 4 mm wide and notched, suggesting left atrial enlargement. The P wave is difficult to see in V1.

Evidence for Ventricular Hypertrophy

LVH: The sum of the S wave in V1 (6 mm) and the R wave in V6 (6 mm) is 12 mm. There is no evidence of left ventricular hypertrophy by voltage criteria. In fact, the voltage is low in both the limb leads and the chest leads, although it does not meet strict criteria for low voltage.

RVH: The QRS axis is in the normal quadrant. There is no evidence for right ventricular hypertrophy.

R-Wave Progression

The R waves do not grow very much from V1 to V3, and the QRS complex does not become positive until V5. Therefore, there is poor R-wave progression.

Evidence of Ischemia or Infarction

Anterior leads: There is poor R-wave progression. The T waves are flat in V1 to V3, and the T waves are inverted in V4 to V6 and I and aVL, consistent with anterolateral ischemia or subendocardial infarction.

Inferior leads: There are no Q waves in the inferior leads. The T waves are flat in II, and the ST segment in aVF is mildly depressed. These changes are suggestive of, but not diagnostic for, ischemia.

Summary

Sinus bradycardia at 50 bpm with first-degree AV block, one pause due to sinus exit block
Intervals: 0.28/0.08/0.44
QRS axis: +15 degrees
Tendency to low voltage and possible left atrial enlargement
Poor R-wave progression consistent with anteroseptal MI, clockwise rotation, or lead placement
T-wave inversion in V4 to V6, I, and aVL consistent with anterolateral ischemia or subendocardial infarction

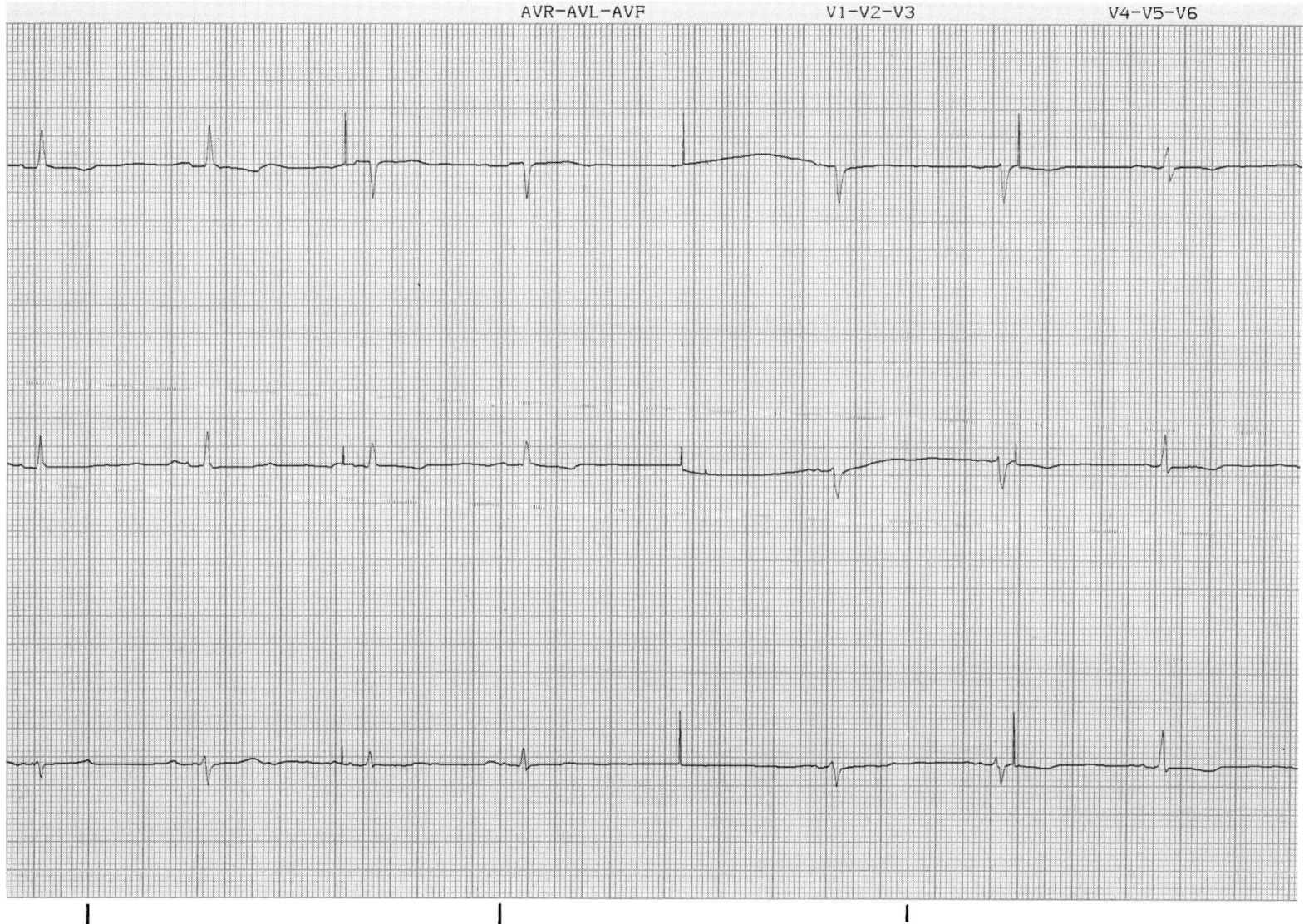

CASE 9

Rate and Rhythm

There is a P wave preceding each QRS complex, and the rhythm is normal sinus rhythm.

The heart rate is about 100 beats per minute.

Intervals

PR interval: 0.20s
QRS duration: 0.12s
QT interval: 0.36s

The QRS duration appears prolonged, but closer examination reveals that the QRS upstrokes slur up from the PR segment, most obviously in I and aVL. This is an example of preexcitation, and the slurred QRS upstrokes are delta waves. This is a tracing from a patient with Wolff-Parkinson-White syndrome.

QRS Axis

The QRS complex is positive in lead I and negative in lead aVF, so the QRS axis is in the leftward axis quadrant. The isoelectric lead is between II and aVR, so the QRS axis is −45 degrees. This is left axis deviation.

Evidence for Atrial Enlargement

In lead II, the P wave is wider than 2.5 mm and is notched. In V1, the P wave is biphasic, and the terminal component is wider than 1 mm. Thus there is left atrial enlargement.

Evidence for Ventricular Hypertrophy

LVH: The sum of the S wave in V1 (9 mm) and the R wave in V6 (11 mm) is 20 mm. There is no evidence of left ventricular hypertrophy by voltage criteria.
RVH: There is left axis deviation, and there is no evidence for right ventricular hypertrophy.

R-Wave Progression

The R waves do not grow very well from V1 to V4, and the QRS complex does not become positive until V5. Thus there is poor R-wave progression.

Evidence of Ischemia or Infarction

There are Q waves in II, III, and aVF that look like evidence of an inferior MI. In this case, however, they are due to Wolff-Parkinson-White syndrome.

Summary

Normal sinus rhythm at 100 bpm
Intervals: 0.20/0.12/0.36
QRS axis: −45 degrees
Delta waves consistent with preexcitation
Left axis deviation
Q waves in II, III, and aVF due to Wolff-Parkinson-White syndrome

CASE 9 • 81

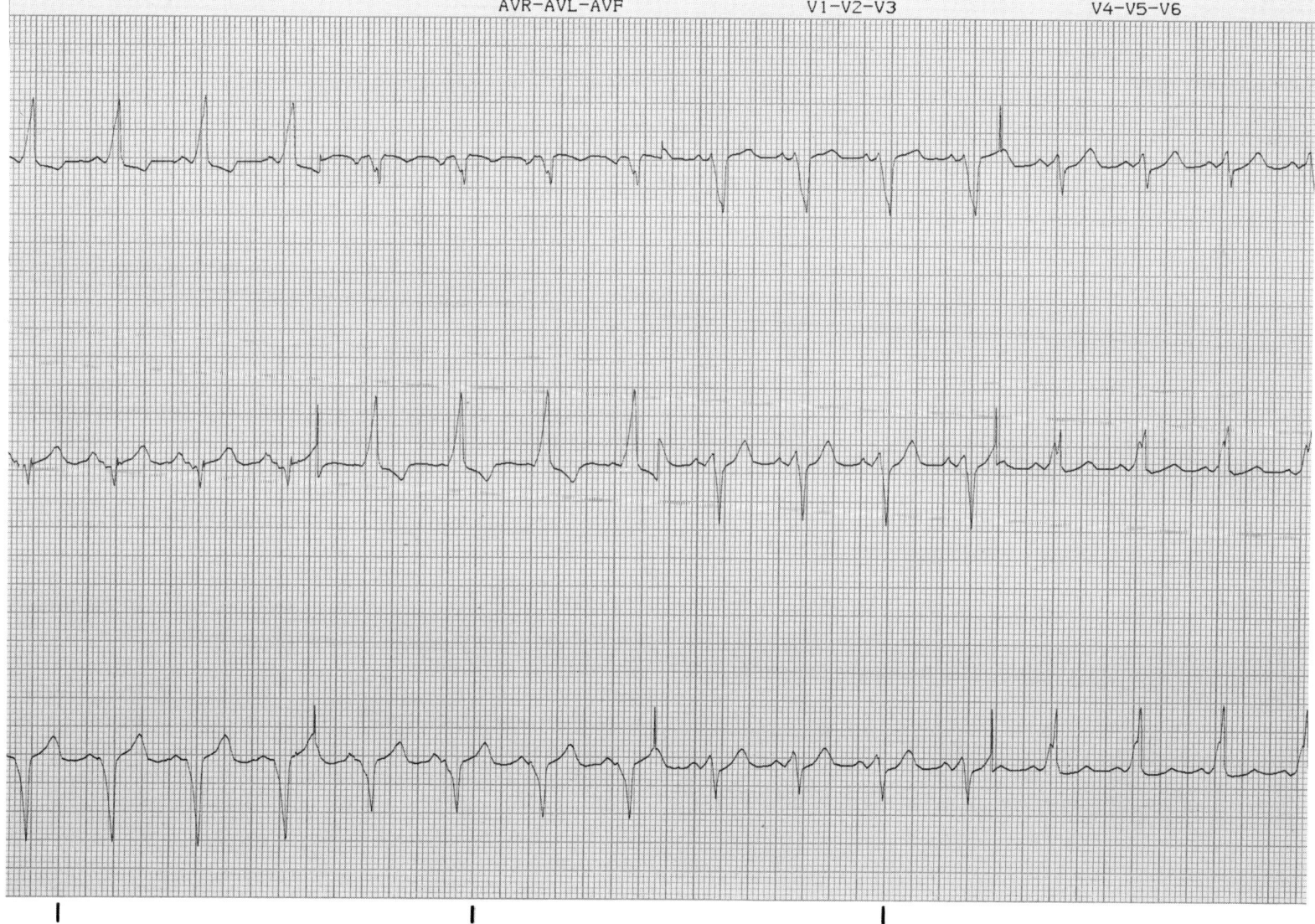

CASE 10

Rate and Rhythm

This is a regular rhythm, but P waves are not apparent. The QRS duration is prolonged to 0.10 s, but not more, so this is a narrow complex tachycardia. The rhythm is paroxysmal atrial tachycardia.

The heart rate is about 170 beats per minute.

Intervals

PR interval: Not applicable (n.a.)
QRS duration: 0.10s
QT interval: 0.28s

There are no visible P waves, so we cannot read a PR interval. The QRS duration is prolonged, but not long enough for a bundle-branch block. The QRS appearance in V1 looks like a right bundle-branch block, so this is an incomplete right bundle-branch block, or an interventricular conduction delay.

QRS Axis

The QRS complex looks isoelectric in many of the leads, making it difficult to determine the axis. This is an example of indeterminate axis.

Evidence for Atrial Enlargement

There are no P waves, so we cannot assess for atrial enlargment.

Evidence for Ventricular Hypertrophy

There is an incomplete right bundle-branch block, so we cannot assess for evidence of ventricular hypertrophy.

R-Wave Progression

The R waves grow from V1 to V6, and the QRS complex becomes mostly positive in leads V3 and V4. Thus there is normal R-wave progression.

Evidence of Ischemia or Infarction

Anterior leads: The R-wave progression is normal. There are downsloping ST-segment depressions in leads V2 and V3 that may indicate anterior ischemia or subendocardial infarction.
Inferior leads: There are no specific changes of inferior ischemia or infarction.
ST-T waves: There are ST-T wave changes from the incomplete right bundle-branch block.

Summary

Paroxysmal atrial tachycardia at 170 bpm
Intervals: n.a./0.10/0.28
QRS axis: indeterminate
Incomplete right bundle-branch block (or interventricular conduction delay)
Downsloping ST-segment depressions in V2 and V3 consistent with anterior ischemia or subendocardial infarction

CASE 10

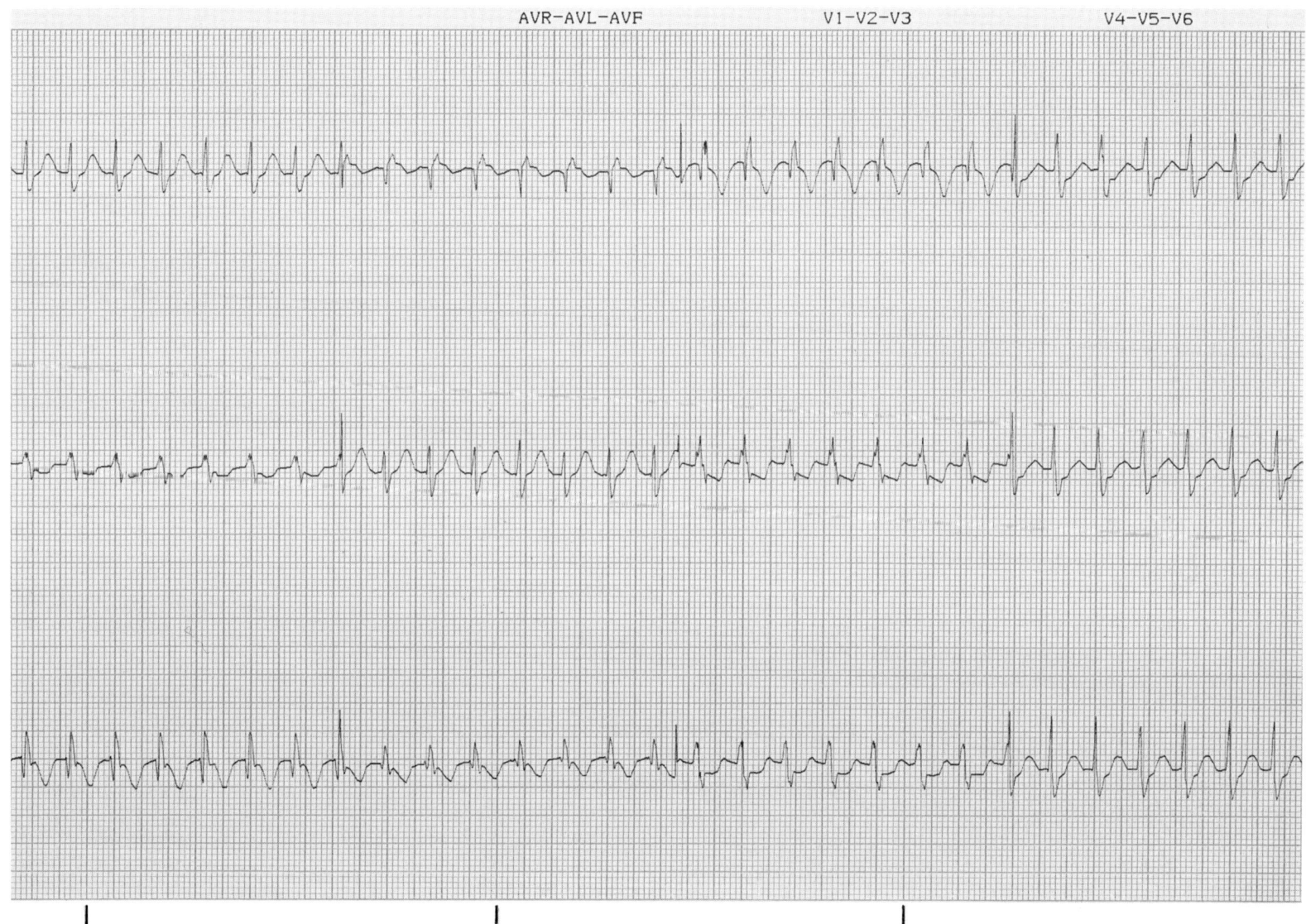

CASE 11

Rate and Rhythm

There is a P wave preceding each QRS complex, and the rhythm is normal sinus rhythm.

The heart rate is about 70 to 80 beats per minute. The heart rate varies slightly during the tracing.

Intervals

PR interval: 0.16s
QRS duration: 0.08s
QT interval: 0.40s

QRS Axis

The QRS complex is positive in lead I and negative in lead aVF, so the QRS axis is in the leftward quadrant. The isoelectric lead is II, so the QRS axis is −30 degrees. This is left axis deviation.

Evidence for Atrial Enlargement

In lead II, the P waves are notched and widened to 3 mm. In lead V1, the P waves are biphasic, with the terminal part wider than 1 mm. Thus there is left atrial enlargement.

Evidence for Ventricular Hypertrophy

LVH: The sum of the S wave in V1 (10 mm) and the R wave in V5 (17 mm) is 27 mm. This does not meet voltage criteria for left ventricular hypertrophy.

RVH: The QRS axis is in the leftward quadrant. There is no evidence for right ventricular hypertrophy.

R-Wave Progression

There is a tall R wave in V1, and the QRS is mostly positive from V2 on. Thus there is R-wave progression that is "too good." The possibilities in this tracing are counterclockwise rotation and posterior MI.

Evidence of Ischemia or Infarction

Anterior leads: There is horizontal to upsloping ST-segment depression in V2 and V3, but this is not specific for ischemia.
Inferior leads: There are Q waves in II, III, and aVF indicating an inferior MI. The ST segments are elevated in the same leads, consistent with acute inferior injury, so we know the MI is acute.
Posterior changes: In the setting of an acute inferior MI, the tall R waves seen in V1 and V2 may be interpreted as indicative of possible posterior MI.

Summary

Normal sinus rhythm at 70 to 80 bpm
Intervals: 0.16/0.08/0.40
QRS axis: −30 degrees
Left axis deviation consistent with left anterior hemiblock
ST-segment elevation and Q waves in II, III, and aVF consistent with acute inferior MI
Tall R waves in V1 and V2 consistent with posterior MI

CASE 11

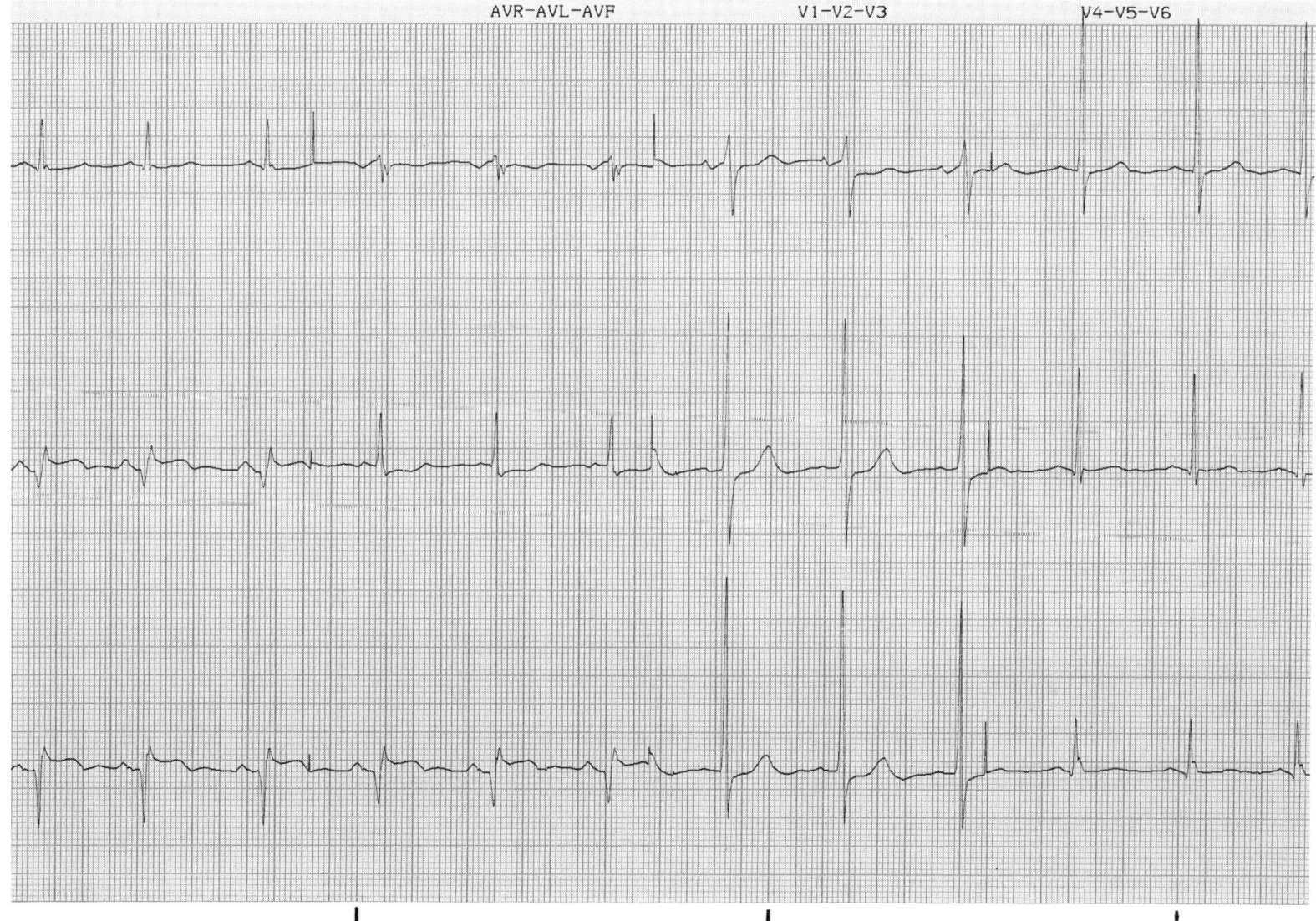

CASE 12

Rate and Rhythm

There is a P wave preceding each QRS complex, and the rhythm is normal sinus rhythm.

The heart rate is about 75 beats per minute.

Intervals

PR interval: 0.16s
QRS duration: 0.08s
QT interval: 0.48s

The QT interval is prolonged for rate.

QRS Axis

The QRS complex is positive in lead I and close to isoelectric in leads II and aVF, so the QRS axis is between 0 and −30 degrees, so it is about −15 degrees.

Evidence for Atrial Enlargement

There is no evidence of atrial enlargment.

Evidence for Ventricular Hypertrophy

LVH: The sum of the S wave in V1 (7 mm) and the R wave in V5 (18 mm) is 25 mm. There is no evidence of left ventricular hypertrophy by voltage criteria.

RVH: The QRS axis is just in the leftward quadrant. There is no evidence for right ventricular hypertrophy.

R-Wave Progression

The R waves grow from V1 to V5, and the QRS becomes mostly positive at V3. Thus there is normal R-wave progression.

Evidence of Ischemia or Infarction

Anterior leads: There is normal R-wave progression. There is T-wave inversion in leads V2 to V6 and I and aVL, consistent with anterior and lateral ischemia or subendocardial infarction.

Inferior leads: The T waves are inverted in II and flat in aVF. These changes are suggestive of, but not diagnostic for, inferior ischemia.

The QT interval is prolonged for rate, consistent with ischemia, electrolyte abnormality, or drug effect.

Summary

Normal sinus rhythm at 75 bpm
Intervals: 0.16/0.08/0.48
QRS axis: −15 degrees
T-wave inversions in leads V2 to V6, I, and aVL consistent with anterior and lateral ischemia or subendocardial infarction
Nonspecific ST-T wave abnormalities in inferior leads

CASE 12 □ 87

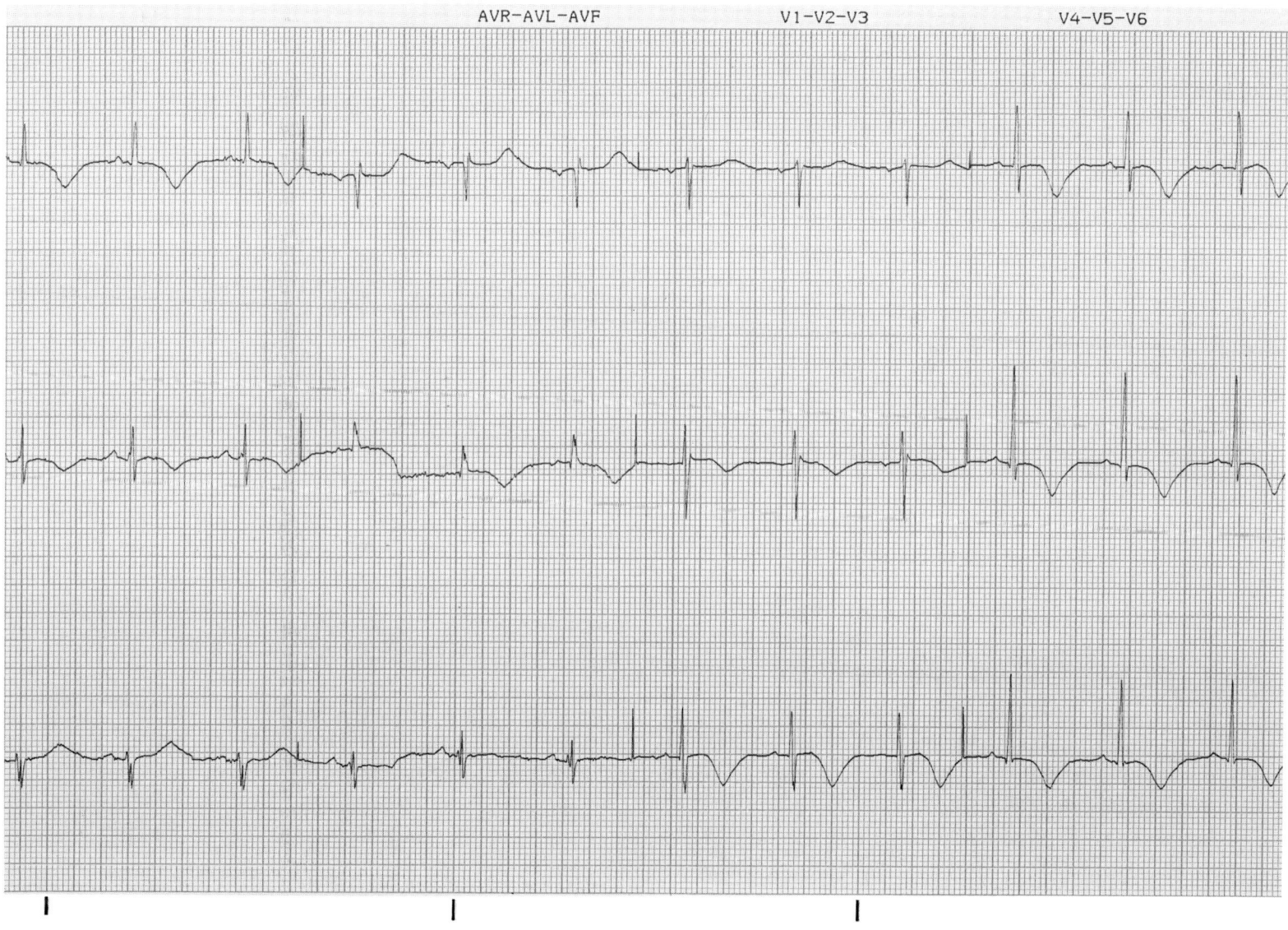

CASE 13

Rate and Rhythm

There is a P wave preceding each QRS complex, and the rhythm is sinus rhythm.

The heart rate is about 55 beats per minute. Because it is less than 60 beats per minute, this is sinus bradycardia.

Intervals

PR interval: 0.16s
QRS duration: 0.06s
QT interval: 0.32s

QRS Axis

The QRS complex is positive in lead I and positive in lead aVF, so the QRS axis is in the normal quadrant. The isoelectric lead is aVL, so the QRS axis is +60 degrees.

Evidence for Atrial Enlargement

There is no evidence for atrial enlargement.

Evidence for Ventricular Hypertrophy

LVH: The sum of the S wave in V1 (20 mm) and the R wave in V5 (30 mm) is 50 mm. This meets the voltage criteria for left ventricular hypertrophy. Note, however, that there are no associated ST-segment changes in this case. This may be a normal variant in a person younger than 35 years old.

RVH: The QRS axis is in the normal quadrant. There is no evidence for right ventricular hypertrophy.

R-Wave Progression

The R waves grow normally from V1 to V5, and the QRS complex becomes mostly positive in V4. Thus there is normal R-wave progression.

Evidence of Ischemia or Infarction

Anterior leads: There is no evidence for anterior ischemia or infarction.
Inferior leads: There is no evidence for inferior ischemia or infarction.
ST-T waves: The T waves are peaked in the anterior leads, and there is early repolarization in leads V4 to V6 and possibly II and aVF. These are nonspecific changes.

Summary

Sinus bradycardia at 55 bpm
Intervals: 0.16/0.06/0.32
QRS axis: +60 degrees
Left ventricular hypertrophy by voltage criteria.
Nonspecific ST-T wave abnormalities

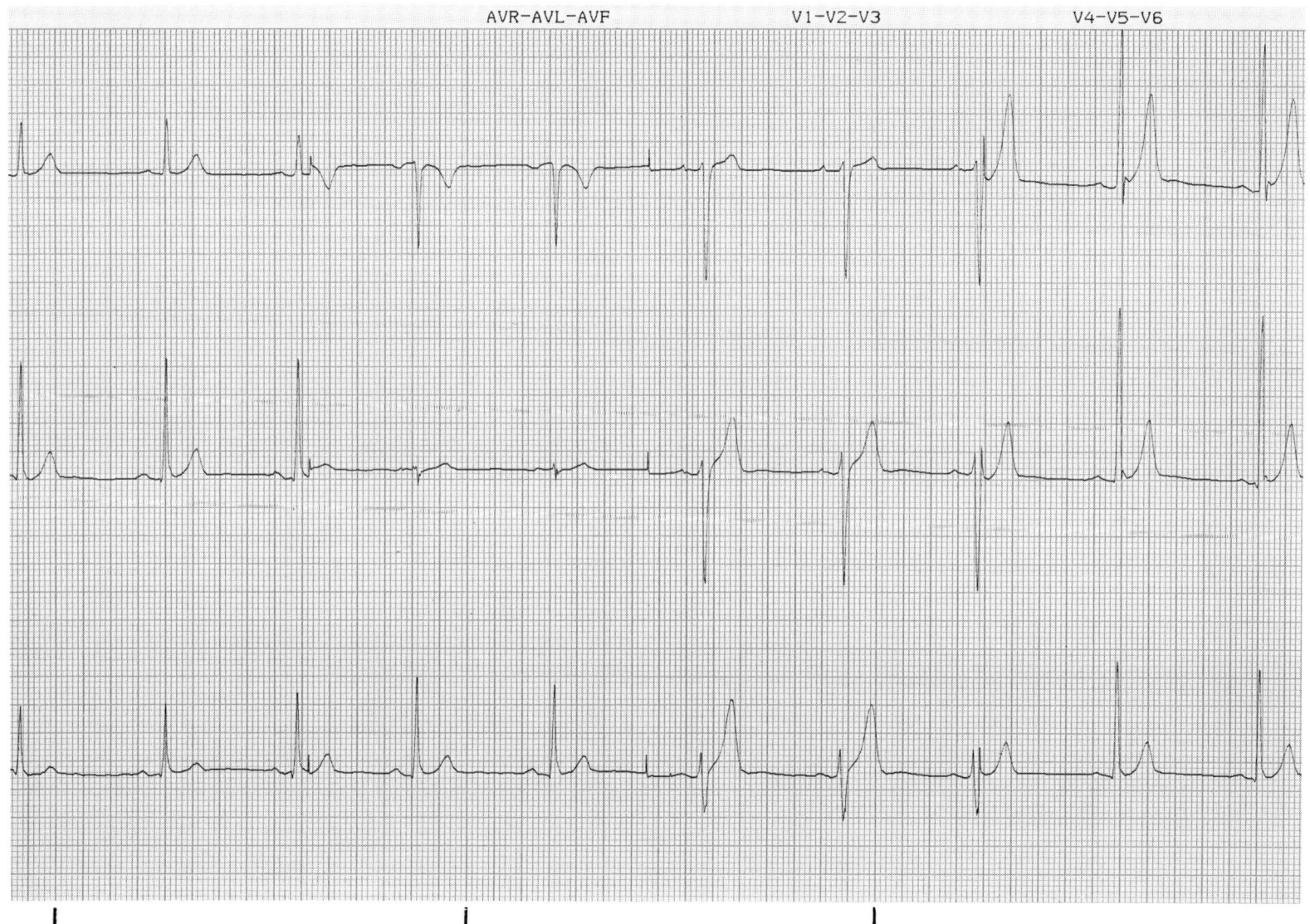

CASE 14

Rate and Rhythm

There is a P wave preceding each QRS complex, and the rhythm is normal sinus rhythm.

The heart rate is about 70 beats per minute.

Intervals

PR interval: 0.12s
QRS duration: 0.06s
QT interval: 0.36s

QRS Axis

The QRS complex is positive in lead I and isoelectric in lead aVF, so the QRS axis is about zero.

Evidence for Atrial Enlargement

There is no evidence for atrial enlargement.

Evidence for Ventricular Hypertrophy

LVH: The sum of the S wave in V1 (12 mm) and the R wave in V5 (14 mm) is 26 mm. There is no evidence of left ventricular hypertrophy by voltage criteria.

RVH: The QRS axis is in the normal quadrant. There is no evidence for right ventricular hypertrophy.

R-Wave Progression

The R waves grow normally from V1 to V5, and the QRS complex becomes mostly positive in V4. Thus there is normal R-wave progression.

Evidence of Ischemia or Infarction

Anterior leads: There is horizontal ST-segment depression in V1 and minimal upsloping ST-segment depression in V2 and V3.

Inferior leads: There is ST-segment elevation in II, III, and aVF, consistent with acute inferior injury. In this setting, the ST-segment depression in V1 may mean posterior injury as well.

Summary

Normal sinus rhythm at 70 bpm
Intervals: 0.12/0.06/0.36
QRS axis: 0 degrees
ST-segment elevation in II, III, and aVF consistent with acute inferior MI
ST-segment depression in V1 consistent with reciprocal change from acute posterior MI

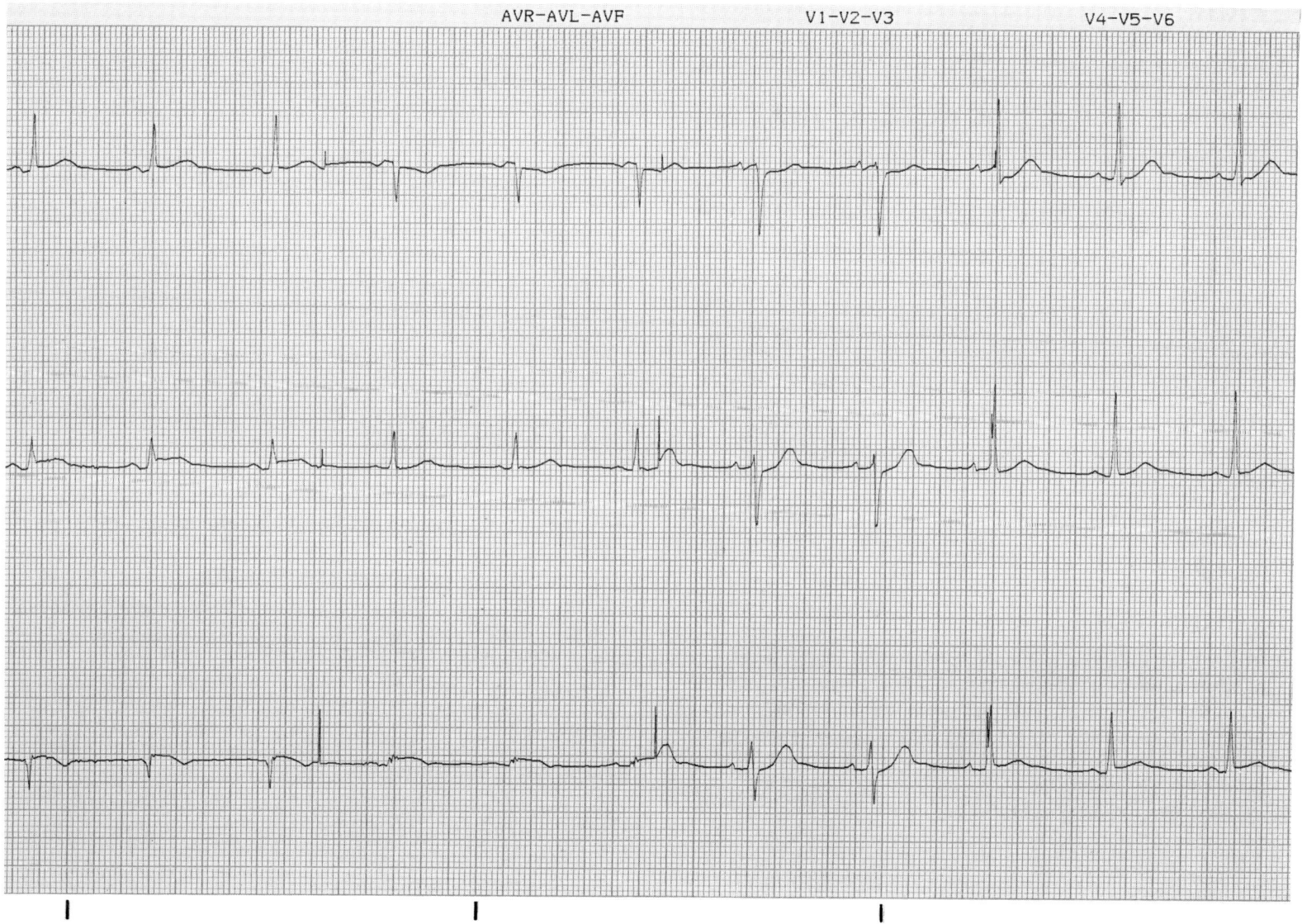

CASE 15

Rate and Rhythm

There is a P wave preceding each QRS complex. However, the P-wave morphology in II, III, and aVF is negative. Normally, P waves are positive in those leads. Thus this rhythm either is due to a low atrial pacemaker or is a junctional rhythm with retrograde P waves.

The heart rate is 90 beats per minute.

Intervals

PR interval: 0.16s
QRS duration: 0.06s
QT interval: 0.48s

The PR interval must be interpreted with caution, since the rhythm is not sinus rhythm. The QT interval is prolonged, which is consistent with ischemia, electrolyte abnormality, or drug effect.

QRS Axis

The QRS complex is positive in lead I and positive in lead aVF, so the QRS axis is in the normal quadrant. Leads III and aVF are closest to isoelectric, so the QRS axis is +15 degrees.

Evidence for Atrial Enlargement

Since atrial depolarization does not originate from the sinus node, we cannot assess for evidence of atrial enlargement.

Evidence for Ventricular Hypertrophy

LVH: The sum of the S wave in V1 (14 mm) and the R wave in V5 (18 mm) is 32 mm. There is no evidence of left ventricular hypertrophy by voltage criteria.
RVH: The QRS axis is in the normal quadrant. There is no evidence for right ventricular hypertrophy.

R-Wave Progression

The R waves grow, although slowly, from V1 to V6. The QRS complex does not become mostly positive until V5. Thus there is poor R-wave progression. In this tracing, the possible explanations are anteroseptal MI, clockwise rotation, and faulty lead placement.

Evidence of Ischemia or Infarction

Anterior leads: There is poor R-wave progression consistent with possible anteroseptal MI. There are no Q waves or ST-segment changes specific for ischemia or infarction.
Inferior leads: There is no specific evidence for ischemia or infarction.
ST-T waves: There is QT prolongation that is consistent with ischemia, electrolyte abnormality, or drug effect.

Summary

Low atrial rhythm at 90 bpm
Intervals: 0.16/0.06/0.48
QRS axis: +15 degrees
QT prolongation consistent with ischemia, electrolyte abnormality, or drug effect

CASE 15 □ 93

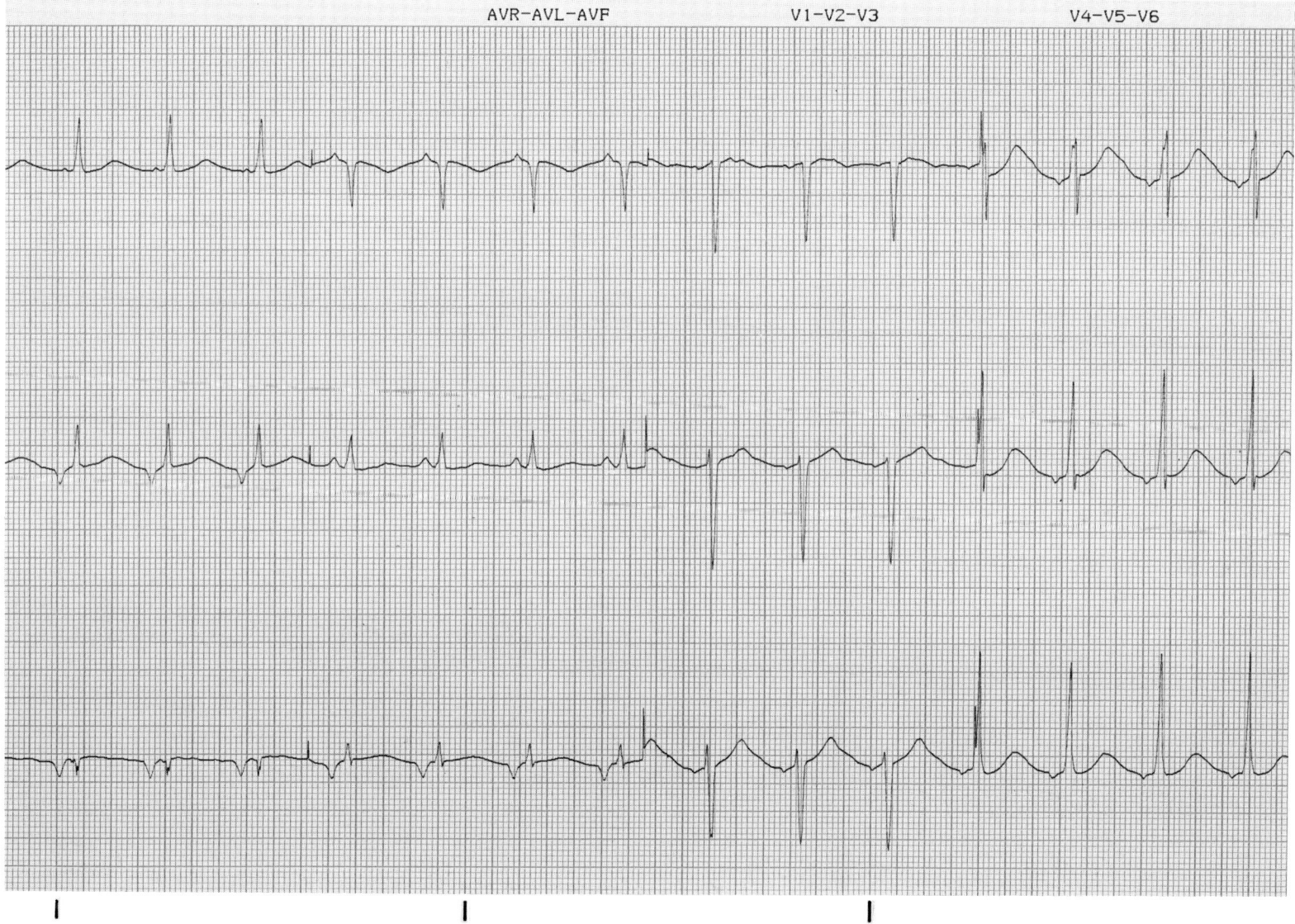

CASE 16

Rate and Rhythm

The rhythm is regular, and the QRS complexes are narrow.

The heart rate is about 150 beats per minute. There are no clear P waves. Examination of leads II, III, and aVF reveals sawtooth-shaped flutter waves. This is atrial flutter with 2:1 conduction.

Intervals

PR interval: Not applicable (n.a.)
QRS duration: 0.08s
QT interval: 0.32s

QRS Axis

The QRS complex is positive in lead I and positive in lead aVF, so the QRS axis is in the normal quadrant. The isoelectric lead is aVL, so the QRS axis is +60 degrees.

Evidence for Atrial Enlargement

In atrial flutter, we cannot assess for evidence of atrial enlargement.

Evidence for Ventricular Hypertrophy

LVH: The sum of the S wave in V1 (7 mm) and the R wave in V6 (11 mm) is 18 mm. There is no evidence of left ventricular hypertrophy by voltage criteria.

RVH: The QRS axis is in the normal quadrant. There is no evidence for right ventricular hypertrophy.

R-Wave Progression

The R waves grow slowly from V1 to V6. The QRS complex does not become mostly positive until V5. Thus there is poor R-wave progression.

Evidence of Ischemia or Infarction

Anterior leads: There is poor R-wave progression. There are no other changes specific for ischemia or infarction.

Inferior leads: There are no changes specific for ischemia or infarction.

Summary

Atrial flutter with 2:1 AV block, ventricular rate 150 bpm
Intervals: n.a./0.08/0.32
QRS axis: +60 degrees
Poor R-wave progression consistent with anteroseptal MI, clockwise rotation, or faulty lead placement

CASE 16

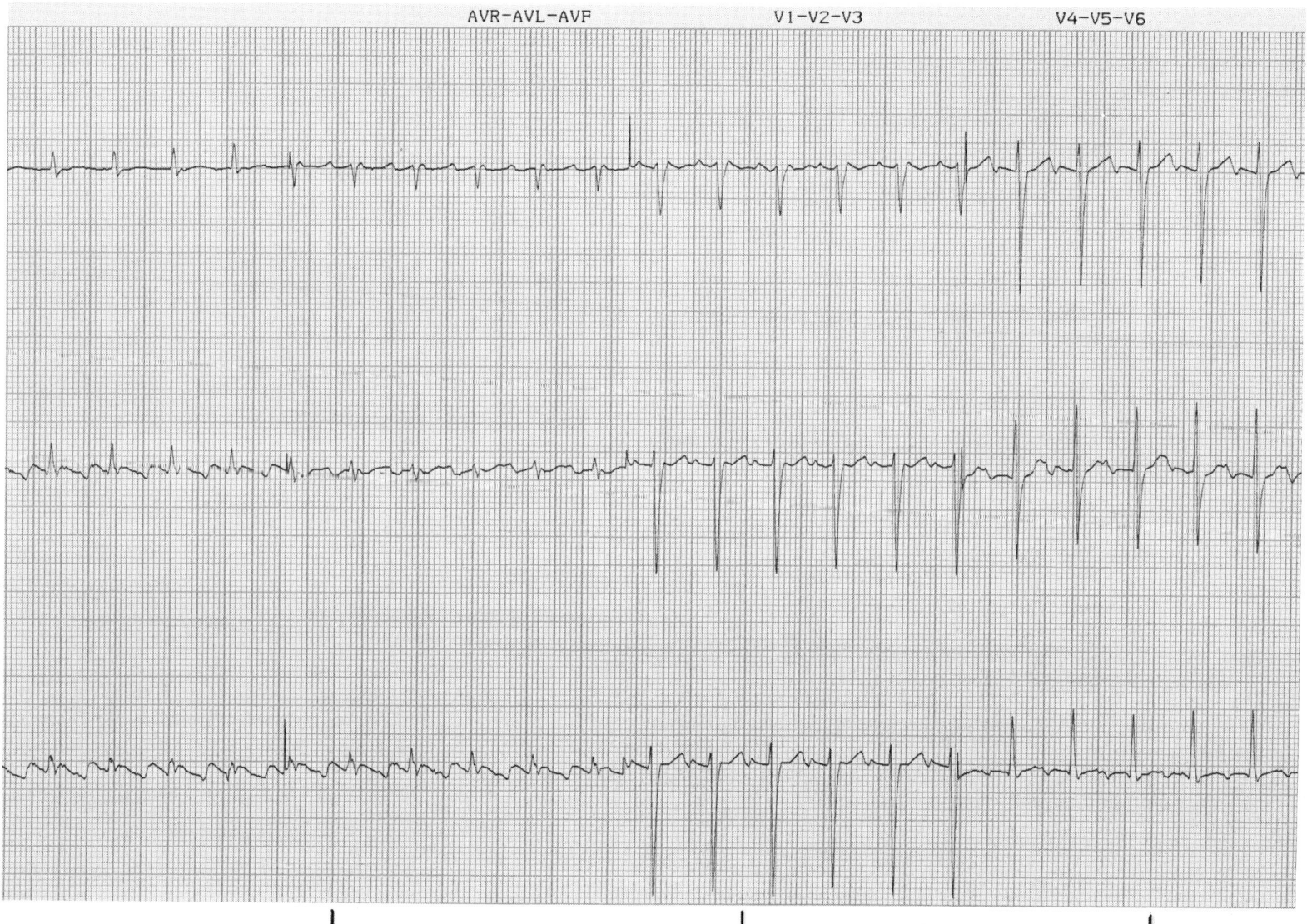

CASE 17

Rate and Rhythm

There is a P wave preceding each QRS complex, and the rhythm is normal sinus rhythm.

The heart rate is about 60 beats per minute.

Intervals

PR interval: 0.16s
QRS duration: 0.08s
QT interval: 0.36s

QRS Axis

The QRS complex is positive in lead I and isoelectric in lead aVF, so the QRS axis is about zero.

Evidence for Atrial Enlargement

In lead II, the P wave is notched and widened to 2.5 mm. This suggests left atrial enlargement. The P wave in lead V1 does not meet criteria, however.

Evidence for Ventricular Hypertrophy

LVH: The sum of the S wave in V1 (16 mm) and the R wave in V6 (6 mm) is 22 mm. There is no evidence of left ventricular hypertrophy by voltage criteria.
RVH: The QRS axis is in the normal quadrant. There is no evidence for right ventricular hypertrophy.

R-Wave Progression

There are Q waves in V1 to V3, and there is no real R-wave growth until V6. Thus there is poor R-wave progression. This is unlikely to be due to faulty lead placement or clockwise rotation alone and suggests an anterior MI.

Evidence of Ischemia or Infarction

Anterior leads: There are Q waves in leads V1 to V3 and poor R-wave progression, consistent with an anterior MI. There is no ST-segment elevation to suggest that it is acute. There are downsloping ST-segment depressions in V4 through V6 and in I and aVL consistent with apicolateral ischemia or subendocardial infarction.
Inferior leads: There are nonspecific ST-T wave abnormalities in the inferior leads.

Summary

Normal sinus rhythm at 60 bpm
Intervals: 0.16/0.08/0.36
QRS axis: 0 degrees
Q waves in V1 to V3, with poor R-wave progression, consistent with anterior MI, and ST-segment depression in V4 to V6, I, and aVL, consistent with apicolateral ischemia or subendocardial infarction
Nonspecific ST-T wave abnormalities in the inferior leads

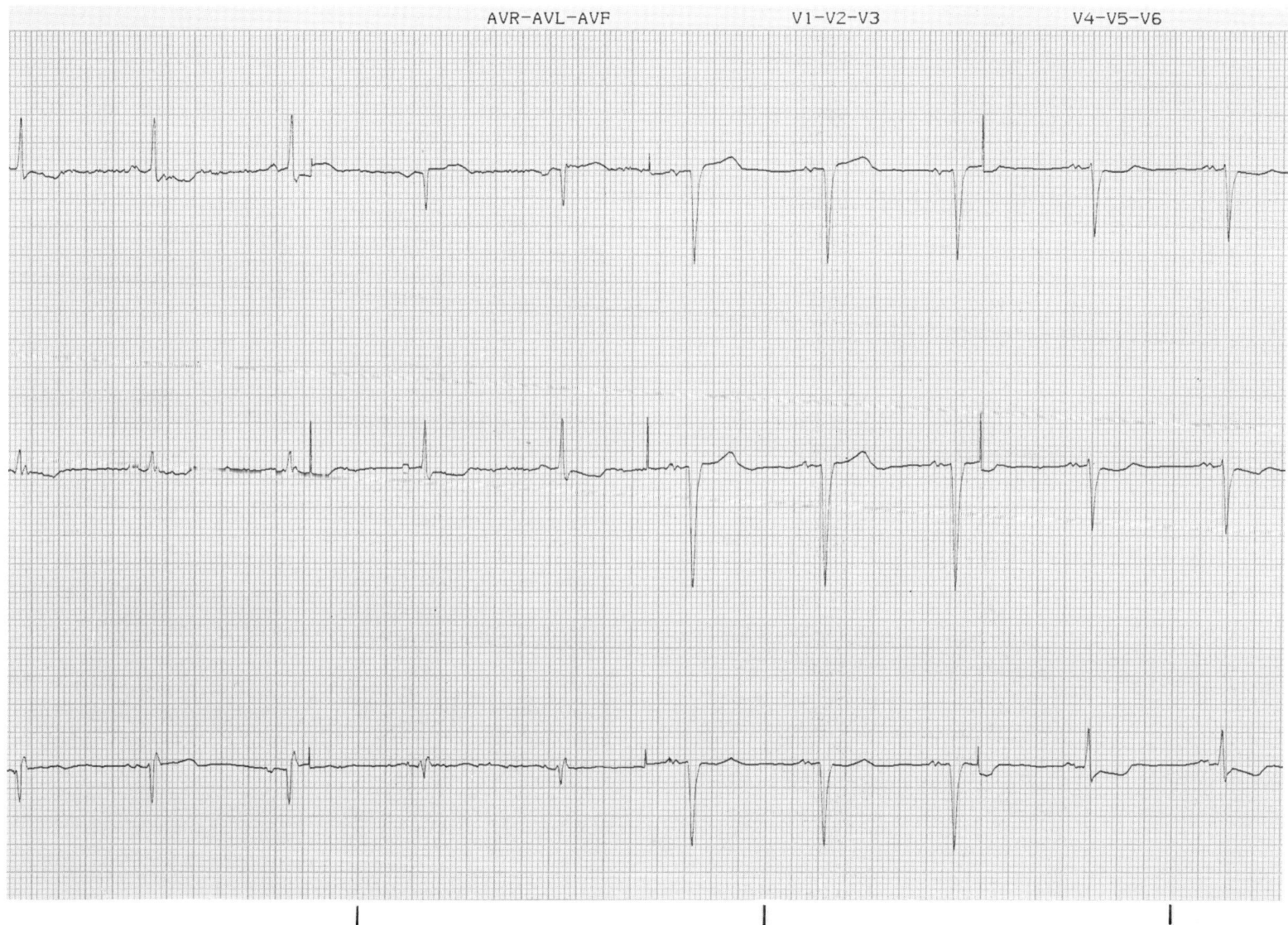

CASE 18

Rate and Rhythm

There is a P wave preceding each QRS complex, and the rhythm is normal sinus rhythm.

The heart rate is about 85 beats per minute.

Intervals

PR interval: 0.16s
QRS duration: 0.08s
QT interval: 0.36s

QRS Axis

The QRS complex is isoelectric in lead I and positive in lead aVF, so the QRS axis is about +90 degrees.

Evidence for Atrial Enlargement

There is no evidence for atrial enlargement.

Evidence for Ventricular Hypertrophy

LVH: The sum of the S wave in V1 (4 mm) and the R wave in V5 (4 mm) is 8 mm. There is no evidence of left ventricular hypertrophy by voltage criteria.
RVH: The QRS axis borders on the rightward quadrant but does not meet the axis criteria for RVH—greater than 100. The R/S ratio in V1 is in fact close to 1 and the R/S ratio in V6 is less than 1, so this tracing does meet the voltage criteria for right ventricular hypertrophy.

R-Wave Progression

The R waves grow slowly, but the QRS complexes never really become positive. Thus there is poor R-wave progression.

Evidence of Ischemia or Infarction

Anterior leads: There are inverted T waves in V1 to V6 and in I and aVL, consistent with anterior and lateral ischemia or subendocardial infarction.
Inferior leads: There are no changes specific for ischemia or infarction in the inferior leads.

Summary

Normal sinus rhythm at 85 bpm
Intervals: 0.16/0.08/0.36
QRS axis: +90 degrees
Poor R-wave progression consistent with clockwise rotation, faulty lead placement, or anterior MI T-wave inversions in V1 to V6, I, and aVL consistent with anterior ischemia or subendocardial infarction

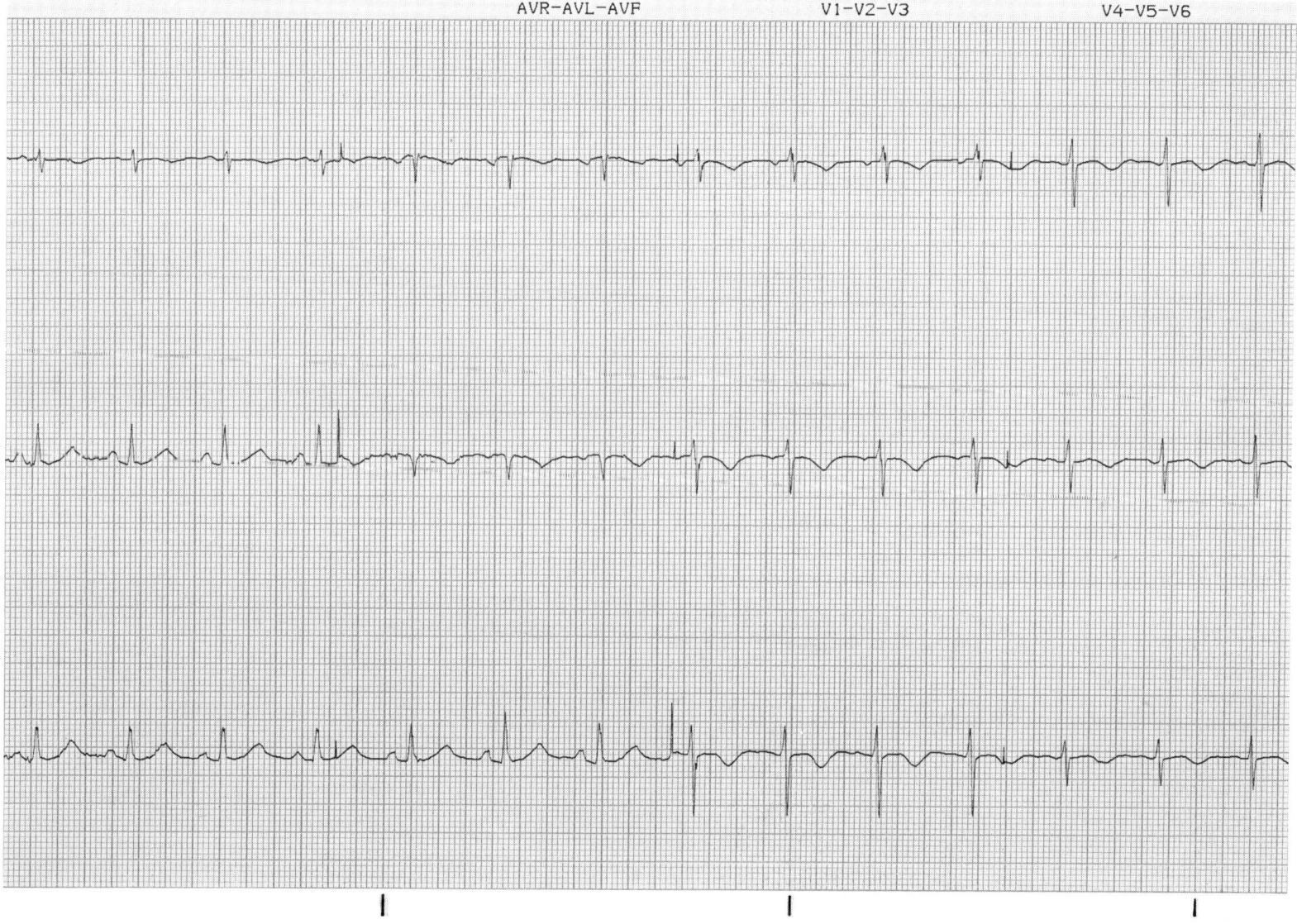

CASE 19

Rate and Rhythm

There is a P wave preceding each QRS complex, and the rhythm is normal sinus rhythm.

The heart rate is about 100 beats per minute. There are occasional wide QRS complexes, which are premature ventricular beats.

Intervals

PR interval: 0.20s
QRS duration: 0.08s
QT interval: 0.40s

QRS Axis

The QRS complex is positive in lead I and negative in lead aVF, so the QRS axis is in the leftward quadrant. The isoelectric lead is II, so the QRS axis is −30 degrees. This is left axis deviation.

Evidence for Atrial Enlargement

In lead II, the P wave is widened to 2.5 mm, suggestive of left atrial enlargement. The P wave in V1 does not appear biphasic with the terminal part wider than 1 mm, however.

Evidence for Ventricular Hypertrophy

LVH: The sum of the S wave in V1 (16 mm) and the R wave in V5 (14 mm) is 30 mm. There is no evidence of left ventricular hypertrophy by voltage criteria.

RVH: The QRS axis is in the leftward quadrant. There is no evidence for right ventricular hypertrophy.

R-Wave Progression

There are Q waves in V1 and V2, and there are no R waves in those leads. Thus there is poor R-wave progression.

Evidence of Ischemia or Infarction

Anterior leads: There are Q waves in V1 and V2 consistent with anteroseptal MI. There is marked ST-segment elevation in leads V1 through V3 and in I and aVL, consistent with acute anterior and lateral injury.

Inferior leads: There are upsloping ST-segment depressions in II, III, and aVF. Because they are upsloping, they are not specific for ischemia.

Summary

Normal sinus rhythm at 100 bpm, with occasional premature ventricular beats
Intervals: 0.20/0.08/0.40
QRS axis: −30 degrees
Left axis deviation consistent with left anterior hemiblock
ST-segment elevation in V1 to V3 and in I and aVL consistent with acute anterolateral MI, with Q waves in V1 and V2
Upsloping ST-segment depressions in II, III, and aVF of unclear significance

CASE 19 □ 101

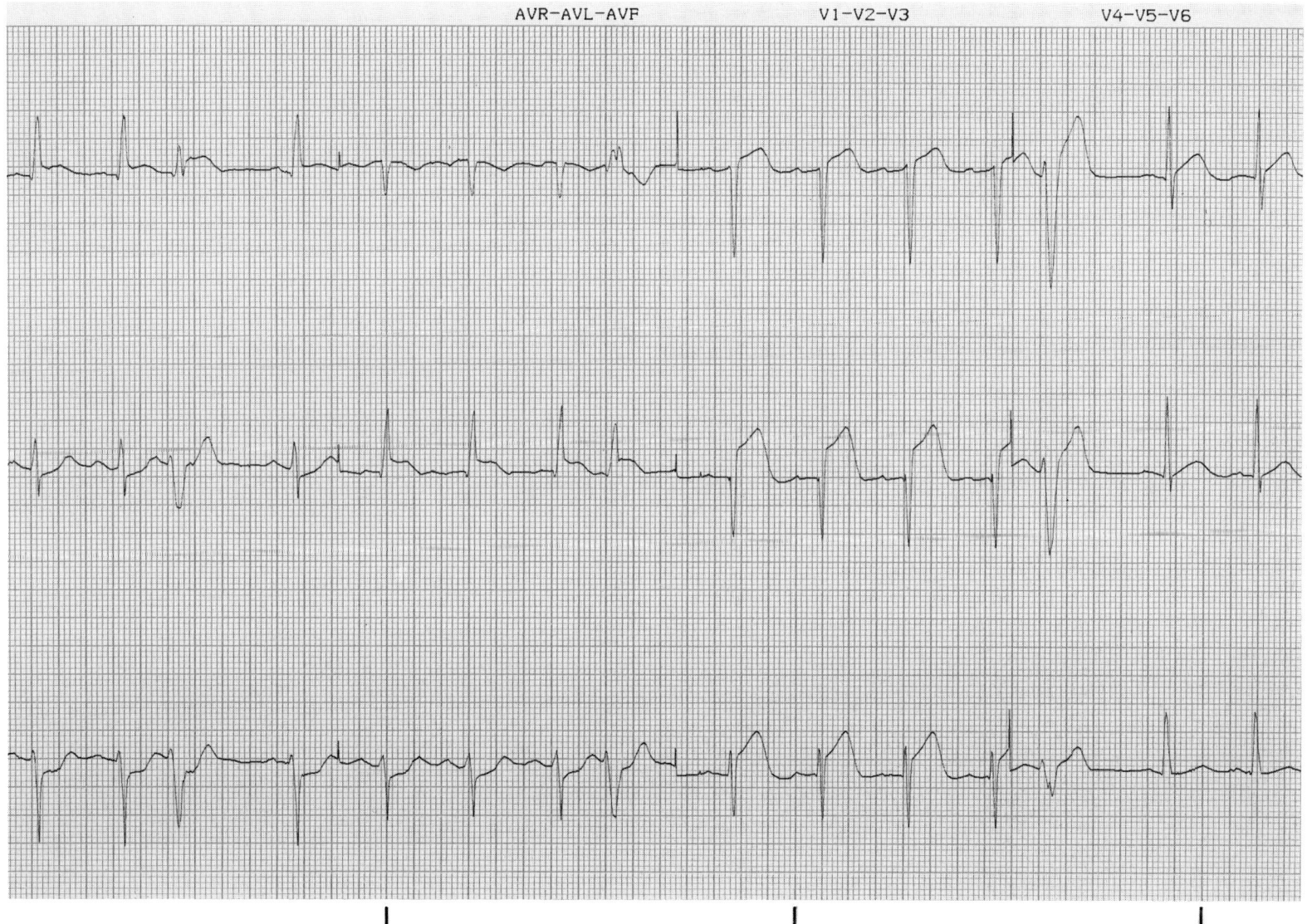

CASE 20

Rate and Rhythm

There is a P wave preceding each QRS complex, and the rhythm is sinus rhythm.

The heart rate is about 100 beats per minute.

Intervals

PR interval: 0.16s
QRS duration: 0.06s
QT interval: 0.36s

QRS Axis

The QRS complex is negative in lead I and positive in lead aVF, so the QRS axis is in the rightward quadrant. There are several leads that look close to isoelectric (aVL, aVR, III, and aVF), so the QRS axis is indeterminate.

Evidence for Atrial Enlargement

In lead II, the P waves are tall and peaked, measuring 3 mm. This suggests right atrial enlargement. The P waves in lead V1 are not clearly visible. However, the findings in lead II are so striking that we could say there is probable right atrial enlargement.

Evidence for Ventricular Hypertrophy

LVH: The sum of the S wave in V1 (0 mm) and the R wave in V5 (9 mm) is 9 mm. There is no evidence of left ventricular hypertrophy by voltage criteria.

RVH: The QRS axis is in the rightward quadrant but is indeterminate. The R/S ratio in V1 is greater than 1, so the tracing meets the voltage criteria for right ventricular hypertrophy.

R-Wave Progression

The R waves grow from V1 to V5, but the QRS complex starts out mostly positive, even in V1. The reasons for the tall R waves in V1 include right ventricular hypertrophy, counterclockwise rotation, and posterior MI.

Evidence of Ischemia or Infarction

Anterior leads: There are nonspecific ST-T wave changes in the anterior leads.

Inferior leads: There are small Q waves in III and aVF that are significant because they are at least 25% of the R-wave height. These Q waves indicate an old inferior MI.

Summary

Normal sinus rhythm at 100 bpm
Intervals: 0.16/0.06/0.36
QRS axis: indeterminate, but with right axis deviation
Probable right atrial enlargement
Voltage criteria for right ventricular hypertrophy
Q waves in II, III, and aVF consistent with old inferior MI

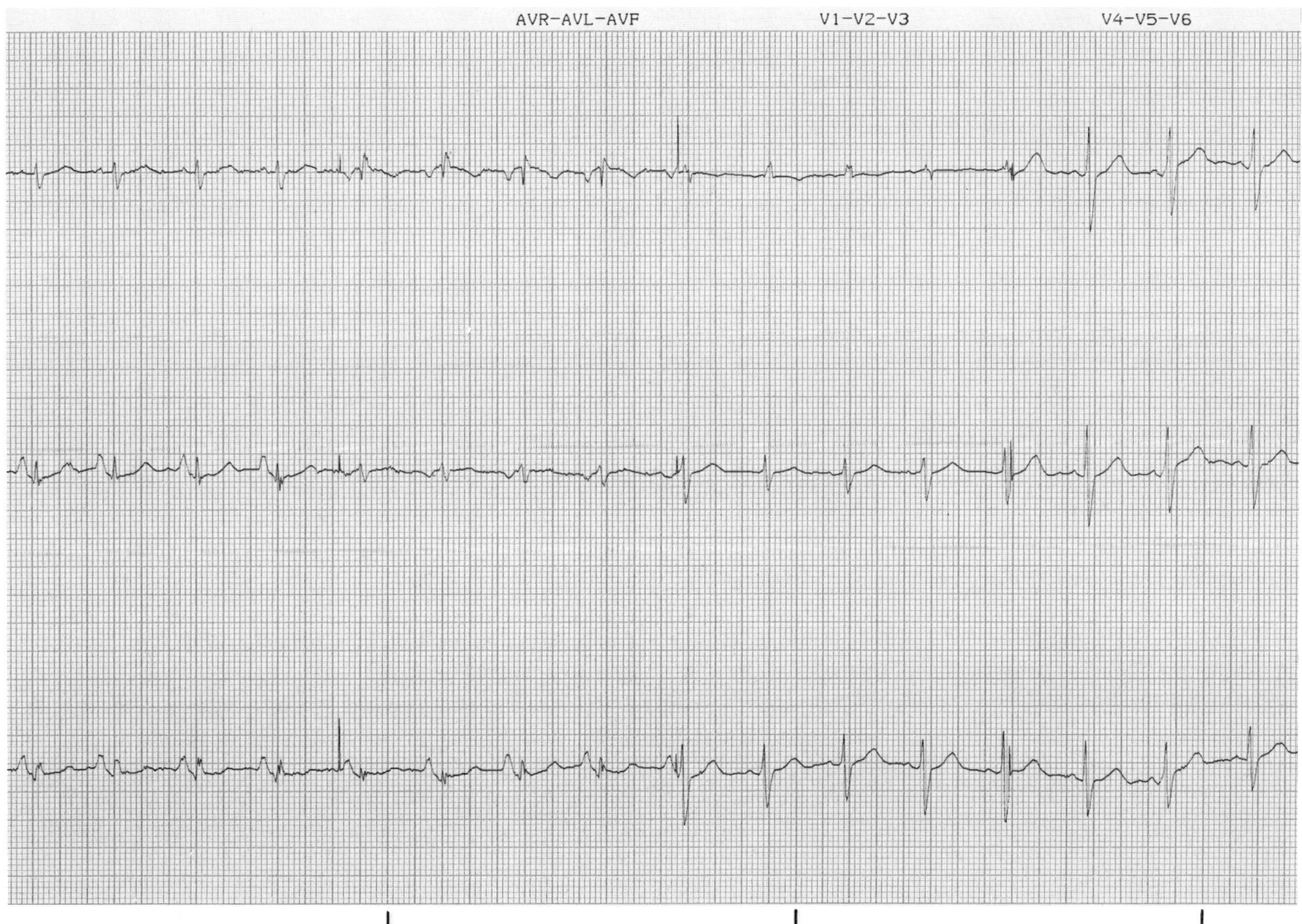

CASE 21

Rate and Rhythm

There is a P wave preceding each QRS complex, and the rhythm is sinus tachycardia.

The heart rate is about 110 beats per minute.

Intervals

PR interval: 0.18s
QRS duration: 0.14s
QT interval: 0.40s

The prolonged QRS duration tells us that there is a bundle-branch block. Examination of lead V1 shows a QRS complex typical of left bundle-branch block.

QRS Axis

The QRS complex is positive in lead I and negative in lead aVF, so the QRS axis is in the leftward quadrant. The isoelectric lead is aVR, so the QRS axis is −60 degrees. This is left axis deviation.

Evidence for Atrial Enlargement

In lead II, the P waves are notched and widened to more than 2.5 mm. In lead V1, the P waves are biphasic, with the terminal part wider than 1 mm. Thus there is left atrial enlargement.

Evidence for Ventricular Hypertrophy

With a left bundle-branch block, we cannot assess criteria for ventricular hypertrophy.

R-Wave Progression

With a left bundle-branch block, we cannot assess R-wave progression.

Evidence of Ischemia or Infarction

With a left bundle-branch block, it is difficult to assess for evidence of ischemia or infarction.

Summary

Sinus tachycardia at 110 bpm
Intervals: 0.18/0.14/0.40
QRS axis: −60 degrees
Left bundle-branch block with left axis deviation
Left atrial enlargement

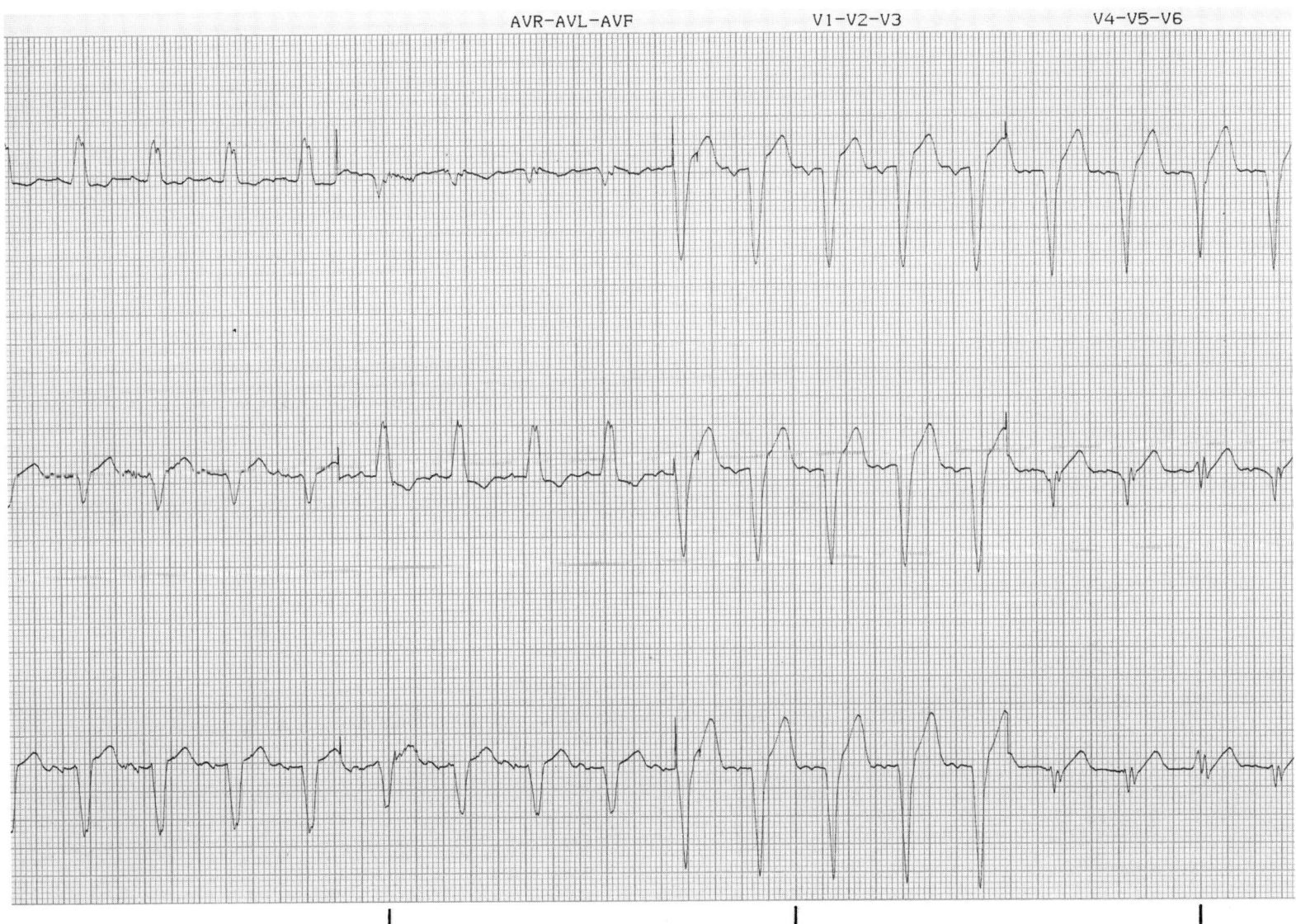

CASE 22

Rate and Rhythm

There is a P wave preceding each QRS complex, and the rhythm is normal sinus rhythm.

The heart rate is about 65 beats per minute.

Intervals

PR interval: 0.12s
QRS duration: 0.10s
QT interval: 0.44s

The QRS duration is prolonged, so there is an incomplete bundle-branch block or an interventricular conduction delay. Since the QRS complex in lead V1 is not typical for either left or right bundle-branch block, we will simply state that there is an interventricular conduction delay.

QRS Axis

The QRS complex is positive in lead I and isoelectric in lead aVF, so the QRS axis is about zero.

Evidence for Atrial Enlargement

There is no evidence for atrial enlargement.

Evidence for Ventricular Hypertrophy

LVH: The sum of the S wave in V1 (16 mm) and the R wave in V5 (20 mm) is 36 mm. Thus there is left ventricular hypertrophy by voltage criteria. Note that there are ST-segment depressions and T-wave inversions in the apical and lateral leads; there are secondary changes from left ventricular hypertrophy.
RVH: The QRS axis is about zero. There is no evidence for right ventricular hypertrophy.

R-Wave Progression

The R waves grow from V1 to V5, and the QRS complex becomes mostly positive in lead V4. Thus there is normal (good) R-wave progression.

Evidence of Ischemia or Infarction

Anterior leads: There is ST-segment depression and T-wave inversion in V4 to V6, I, and aVL consistent with apicolateral ischemia or subendocardial infarction. However, in the setting of left ventricular hypertrophy, these changes are likely to be secondary to left ventricular hypertrophy.
Inferior leads: There are Q waves and ST-segment elevation in leads II, III, and aVF consistent with an acute inferior MI.

Summary

Normal sinus rhythm at 65 bpm
Intervals: 0.12/0.10/0.44
QRS axis: 0 degrees
Interventricular conduction delay
Left ventricular hypertrophy with secondary ST-T wave abnormalities
Q waves and ST-segment elevation in leads II, III, and aVF consistent with acute inferior MI

CASE 22 □ 107

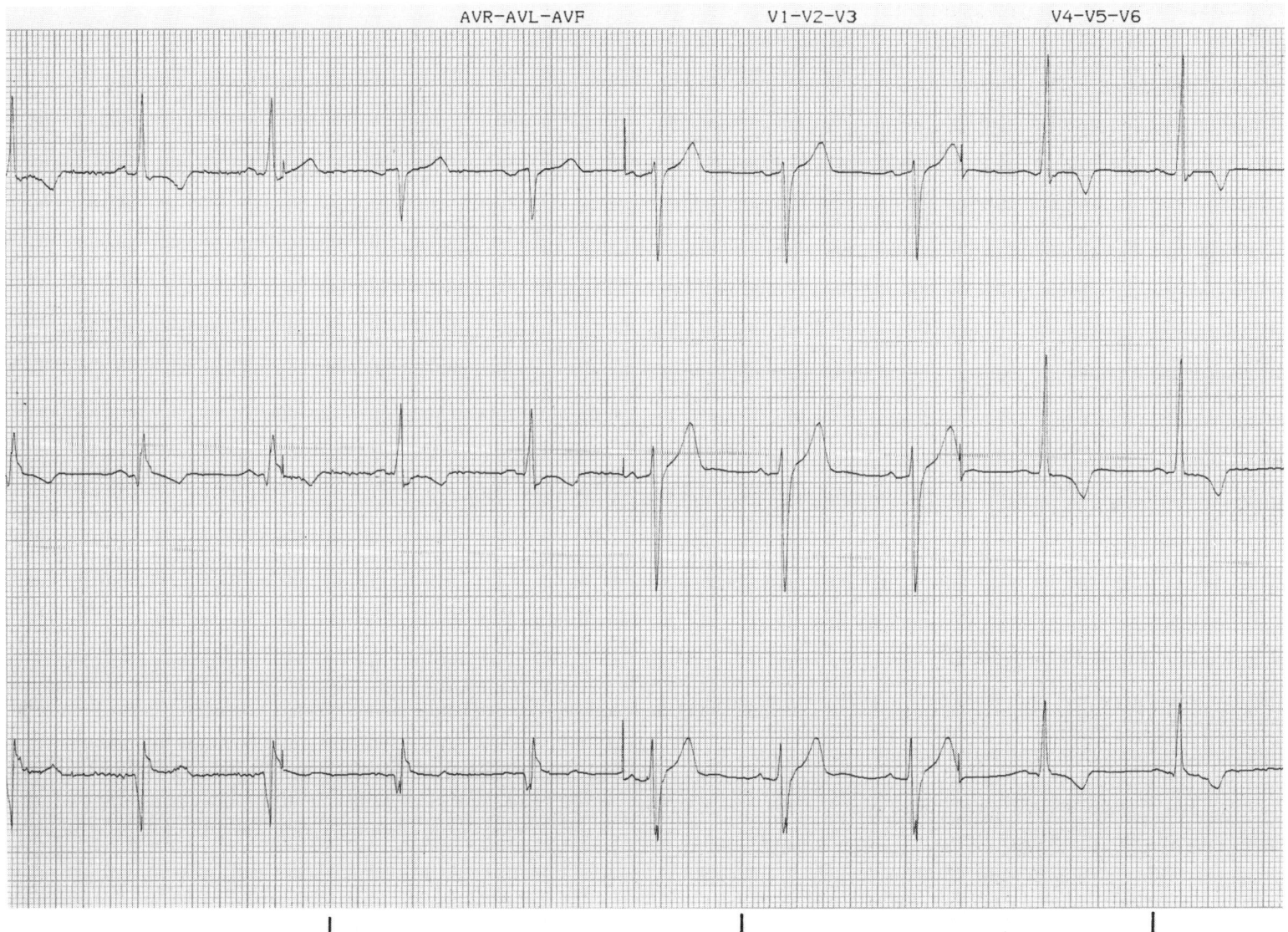

CASE 23

Rate and Rhythm

There are P waves preceding the QRS complexes, and the rhythm is normal sinus rhythm.

The heart rate is about 85 beats per minute. Note that the fourth beat is earlier than expected. It is identical in shape to the other QRS complexes, so it is supraventricular in origin. It is an atrial premature beat.

Intervals

   PR interval: 0.20s
   QRS duration: 0.06s
   QT interval: 0.32s

The PR interval is at the upper limit of normal.

QRS Axis

The QRS complex is positive in lead I and negative in lead aVF, so the QRS axis is in the leftward quadrant. The isoelectric lead is II, so the QRS axis is −30 degrees. This is left axis deviation.

Evidence for Atrial Enlargement

In lead II, the P wave appears wide but is difficult to see. In V1, neither part of the biphasic P wave is greater than 1 mm. Thus this tracing does not meet criteria for atrial enlargement.

Evidence for Ventricular Hypertrophy

LVH: The sum of the S wave in V1 (1 mm) and the R wave in V5 (16 mm) is 17 mm. There is no evidence of left ventricular hypertrophy by voltage criteria.
RVH: The QRS axis is in the leftward quadrant. Thus we cannot diagnose right ventricular hypertrophy.

R-Wave Progression

The R waves start out tall in V1 and grow through V4. The QRS complex is positive in all the precordial leads. The reasons for these tall R waves in V1 and V2 include counterclockwise rotation, posterior MI, and faulty lead placement.

Evidence of Ischemia or Infarction

Anterior leads: There are downsloping ST segments in V1 to V4 that are suggestive of anterior ischemia.
Inferior leads: There are Q waves in II, III, and aVF consistent with an inferior MI. In this setting, the tall R waves in V1 and V2 are likely to be from posterior involvement of the MI.

Summary

Normal sinus rhythm at 85 bpm, with one atrial premature beat
Intervals: 0.20/0.06/0.32
QRS axis: −30 degrees
Left axis deviation consistent with left anterior hemiblock
Q waves in II, III, and aVF with tall R waves in V1 and V2 consistent with inferoposterior MI
Mild ST-segment depression in V1 to V4 consistent with anterior ischemia

CASE 23

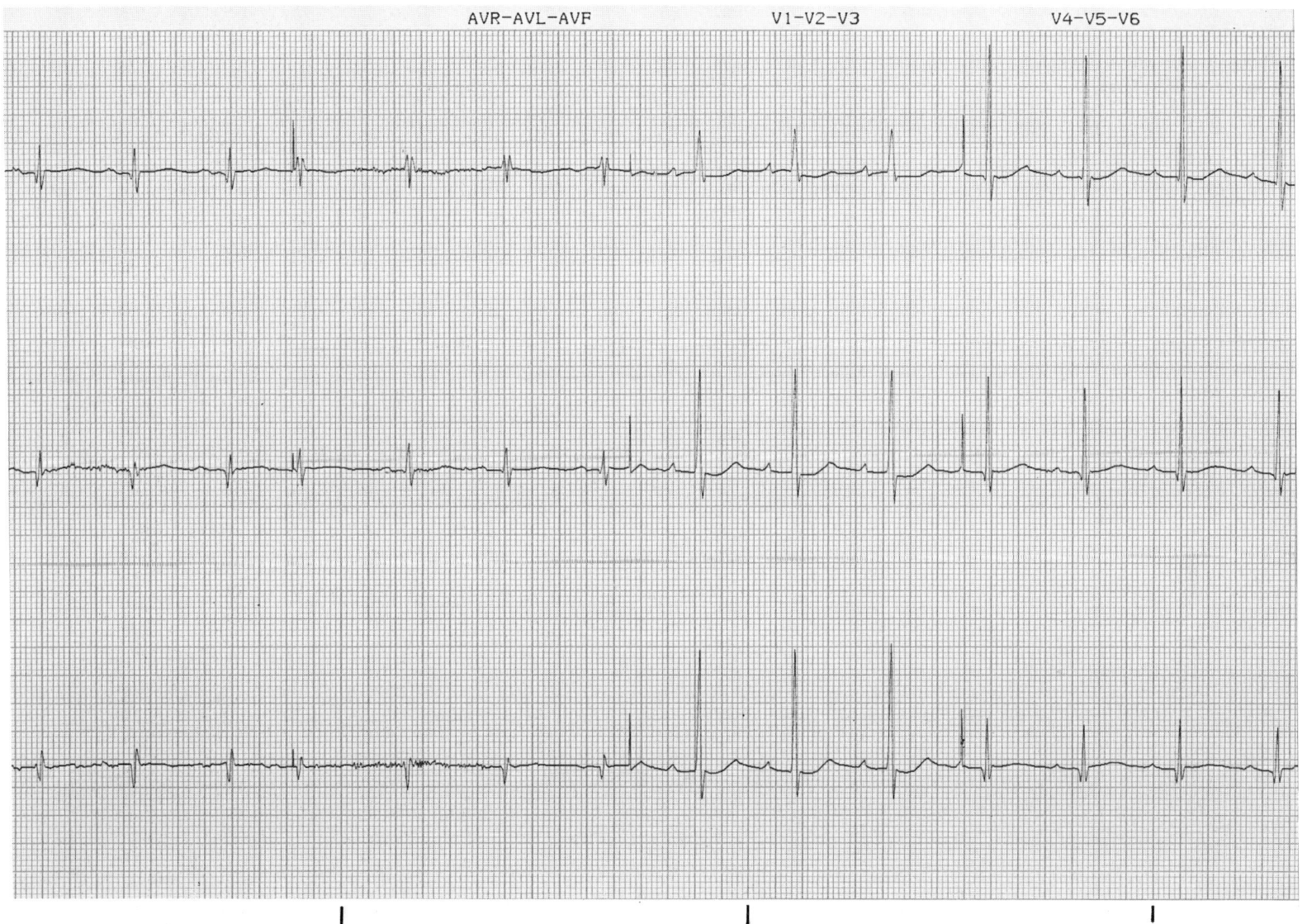

CASE 24

Rate and Rhythm

There is a P wave preceding each QRS complex, and the rhythm is normal sinus rhythm.

The heart rate is about 75 beats per minute.

Intervals

PR interval: 0.12s
QRS duration: 0.06s
QT interval: 0.36s

QRS Axis

The QRS complex is positive in lead I and positive in lead aVF, so the QRS axis is in the normal quadrant. The isoelectric lead is aVL, so the QRS axis is +60 degrees.

Evidence for Atrial Enlargement

There is no evidence for atrial enlargement.

Evidence for Ventricular Hypertrophy

LVH: The sum of the S wave in V1 (5 mm) and the R wave in V6 (5 mm) is 11 mm. There is no evidence of left ventricular hypertrophy by voltage criteria.

RVH: The QRS axis is in the normal quadrant. There is no evidence for right ventricular hypertrophy.

R-Wave Progression

The R waves grow in size from V1 to V6 slowly. The QRS complex does not become mostly positive until V5. Thus there is poor R-wave progression. This is consistent with clockwise rotation or faulty lead placement. While anterior MI is a possibility, the other causes of poor R-wave progression are more likely.

Evidence of Ischemia or Infarction

Anterior leads: There is poor R-wave progression but no other signs of ischemia or infarction.
Inferior leads: There is no evidence of ischemia or infarction.

Summary

Normal sinus rhythm at 75 bpm
Intervals: 0.12/0.06/0.36
QRS axis: +60 degrees
Poor R-wave progression consistent with clockwise rotation or faulty lead placement

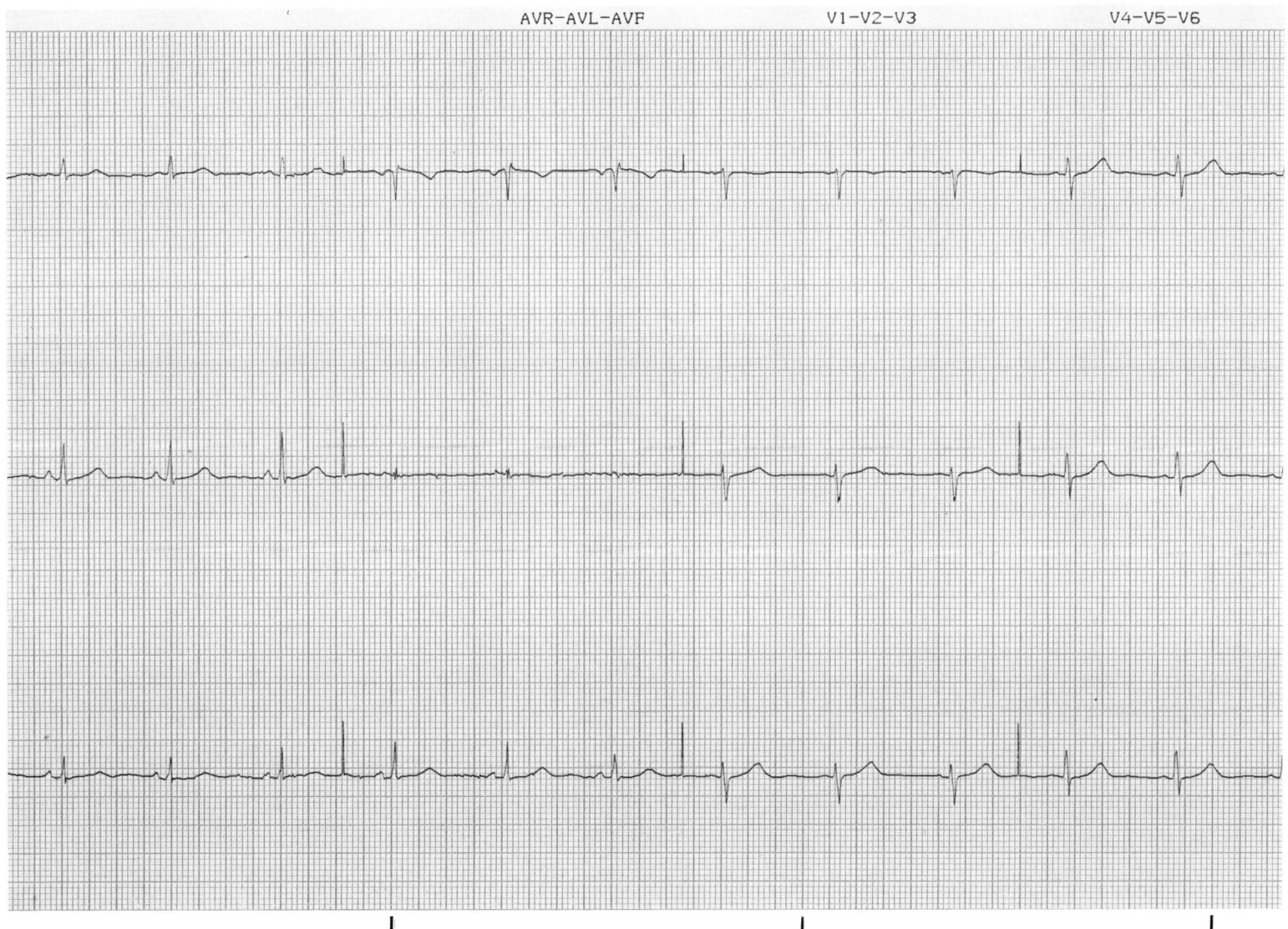

CASE 25

Rate and Rhythm

There is a P wave preceding each QRS complex, and the rhythm is normal sinus rhythm.

The heart rate is about 70 beats per minute.

Intervals

PR interval: 0.16s
QRS duration: 0.08s
QT interval: 0.44s

QRS Axis

The QRS complex is positive in lead I and negative in lead aVF, so the QRS axis is in the leftward quadrant. The isoelectric lead is between II and aVF, so the QRS axis is −15 degrees. This is leftward axis but, strictly speaking, not left axis deviation.

Evidence for Atrial Enlargement

There is no evidence for atrial enlargement.

Evidence for Ventricular Hypertrophy

LVH: The sum of the S wave in V1 (10 mm) and the R wave in V5 (13 mm) is 23 mm. There is no evidence of left ventricular hypertrophy by voltage criteria.

RVH: The QRS axis is in the leftward quadrant. There is no evidence for right ventricular hypertrophy.

R-Wave Progression

The R waves grow in size from V1 to V5, and the QRS complex becomes mostly positive at V4. Thus there is normal (good) R-wave progression.

Evidence of Ischemia or Infarction

Anterior leads: There is no specific evidence of ischemia or infarction. The T waves in V6 are flat, and there are upsloping ST-segment depressions in I and aVL. These are nonspecific changes.

Inferior leads: There are Q waves, ST-segment elevations, and T-wave inversions in III and aVF consistent with an acute inferior MI.

Summary

Normal sinus rhythm at 75 bpm
Intervals: 0.16/0.08/0.44
QRS axis: −15 degrees
Leftward axis
Q waves, ST-segment elevations, and T-wave inversions in leads III and aVF consistent with acute inferior MI

CASE 25 □ 113

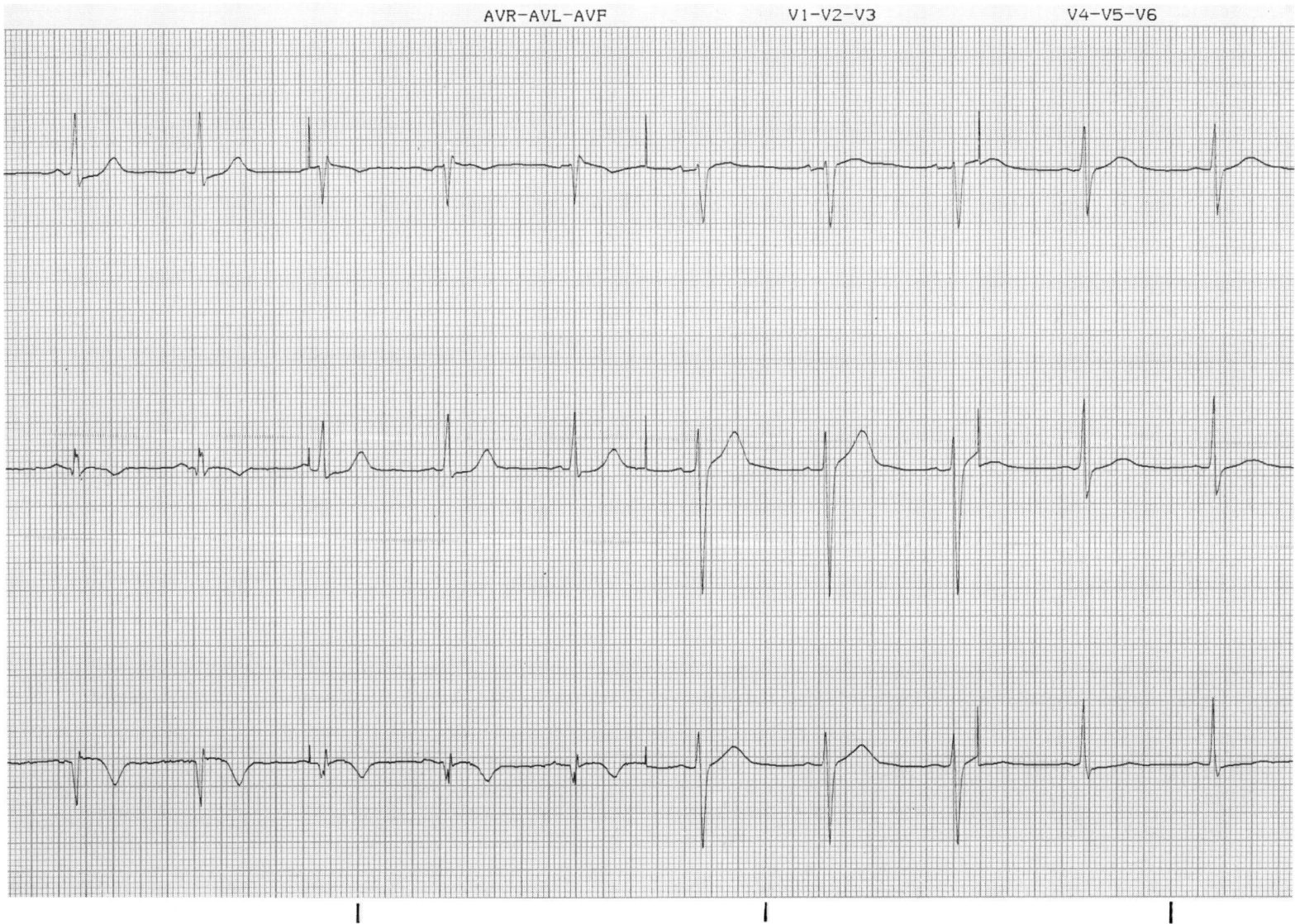

CASE 26

Rate and Rhythm

There is a P wave preceding each QRS complex, and the rhythm is normal sinus rhythm.

The heart rate is about 80 beats per minute.

Intervals

PR interval: 0.20s
QRS duration: 0.10s
QT interval: 0.40s

The PR interval is at the upper limit of normal. The QRS duration is prolonged, indicating an interventricular conduction delay. In V1, the pattern is most consistent with an incomplete left bundle-branch block.

QRS Axis

The QRS complex is isoelectric in lead I and positive in lead aVF, so the QRS axis is about +90 degrees.

Evidence for Atrial Enlargement

In lead II, the P waves are wide, measuring greater than 2.5 mm. In lead V1, the P waves are biphasic, with the terminal part wider than 1 mm. Thus there is left atrial enlargement.

Evidence for Ventricular Hypertrophy

LVH: The sum of the S wave in V1 (11 mm) and the R wave in V5 (13 mm) is 24 mm. There is no evidence of left ventricular hypertrophy by voltage criteria.

RVH: The QRS axis is about +90 degrees. There is no evidence for right ventricular hypertrophy.

R-Wave Progression

The R waves grow from V1 to V5 but do not become mostly positive until V5. Thus there is poor R-wave progression. In this case, it is consistent with the interventricular conduction delay. Clockwise rotation, faulty lead placement, and anterior MI are other possibilities.

Evidence of Ischemia or Infarction

Anterior leads: There are no specific signs of ischemia or infarction.
Inferior leads: There are no specific signs of ischemia or infarction.
ST-T waves: There is ST-segment depression in V5, V6, II, III, and aVF. This is most likely due to the interventricular conduction delay.

Summary

Normal sinus rhythm at 80 bpm
Intervals: 0.20/0.10/0.40
QRS axis: +90 degrees
Interventricular conduction delay (or incomplete left bundle-branch block) with secondary ST-T wave changes
Left atrial enlargement

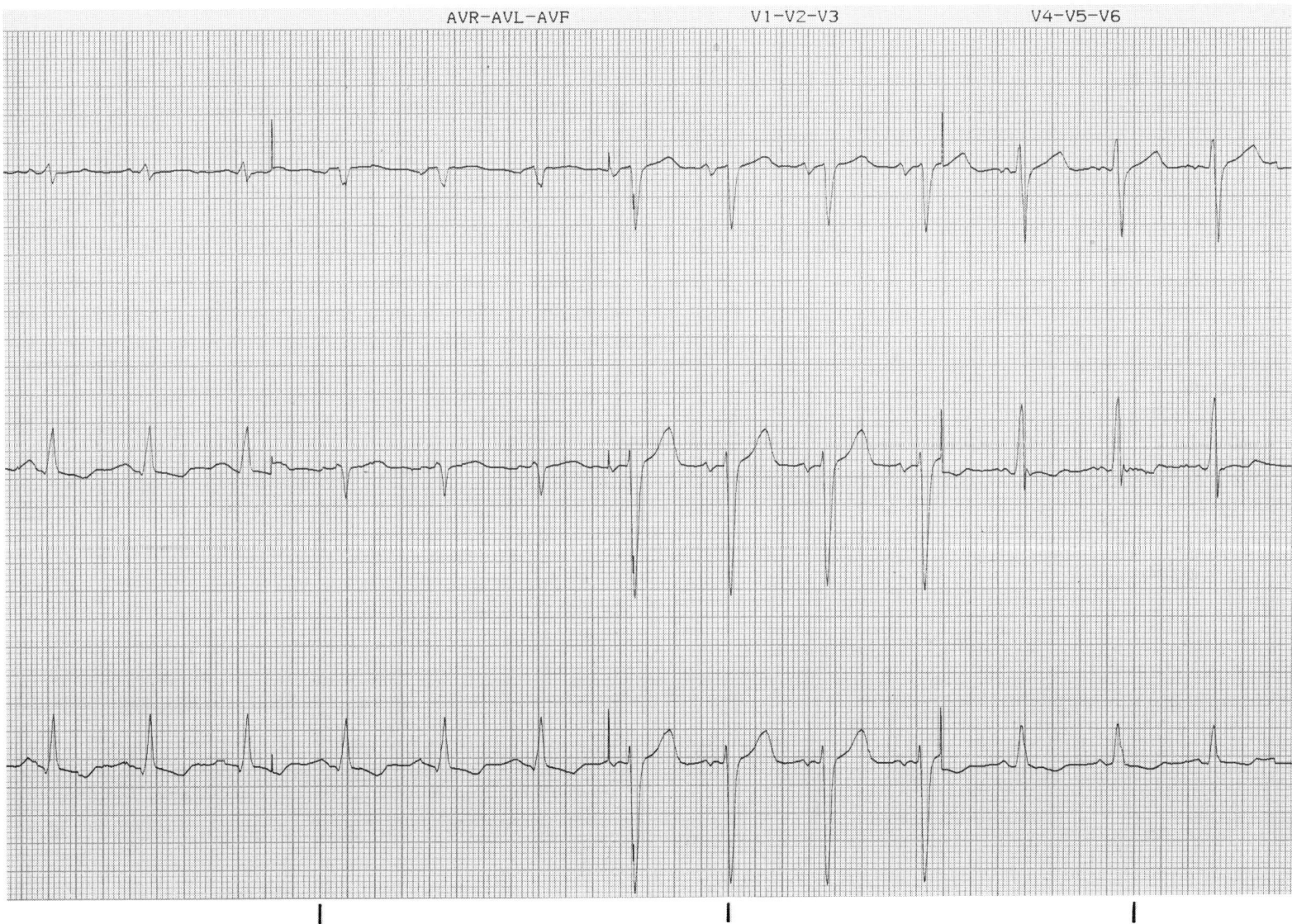

CASE 27

Rate and Rhythm

There is a P wave preceding each QRS complex, and the rhythm is sinus tachycardia.

The heart rate is about 120 beats per minute.

Intervals

PR interval: 0.16s
QRS duration: 0.06s
QT interval: 0.32s

QRS Axis

The QRS complex is negative in lead I and positive in lead aVF, so the QRS axis is in the rightward quadrant. The isoelectric lead is aVR, so the QRS axis is +120 degrees. This is right axis deviation.

Evidence for Atrial Enlargement

In lead II, the P waves are peaked, measuring more than 2.5 mm tall. In lead V1, the P waves are biphasic, with the first part wider than 1 mm. Thus there is right atrial enlargement.

Evidence for Ventricular Hypertrophy

LVH: The sum of the S wave in V1 (0 mm) and the R wave in V5 (5 mm) is 5 mm. There is no evidence of left ventricular hypertrophy.
RVH: The QRS axis is +120 degrees, which meets the axis criterion for right ventricular hypertrophy. The R/S ratio in lead V1 is greater than 1. The R/S ratio in lead V6 is also less than 1. Thus both axis and voltage criteria have been satisfied, and there is right ventricular hypertrophy.

R-Wave Progression

The R waves do not grow across the precordium. The QRS complexes are positive in V1 but not in the other leads. There is poor R-wave progression. In this tracing, it is most likely due to clockwise rotation, faulty lead placement, or chronic obstructive lung disease.

Evidence of Ischemia or Infarction

Anterior leads: There is no specific evidence of ischemia or infarction.
Inferior leads: There is mild ST-segment depression in III and aVF, but these changes are not marked enough to be specific.

Summary

Sinus tachycardia at 120 bpm
Intervals: 0.16/0.06/0.32
QRS axis: +120 degrees
Right axis deviation
Right atrial enlargement
Right ventricular hypertrophy
Poor R-wave progression, most likely due to clockwise rotation, faulty lead placement, or chronic obstructive lung disease, although anterior subendocardial infarction cannot be excluded

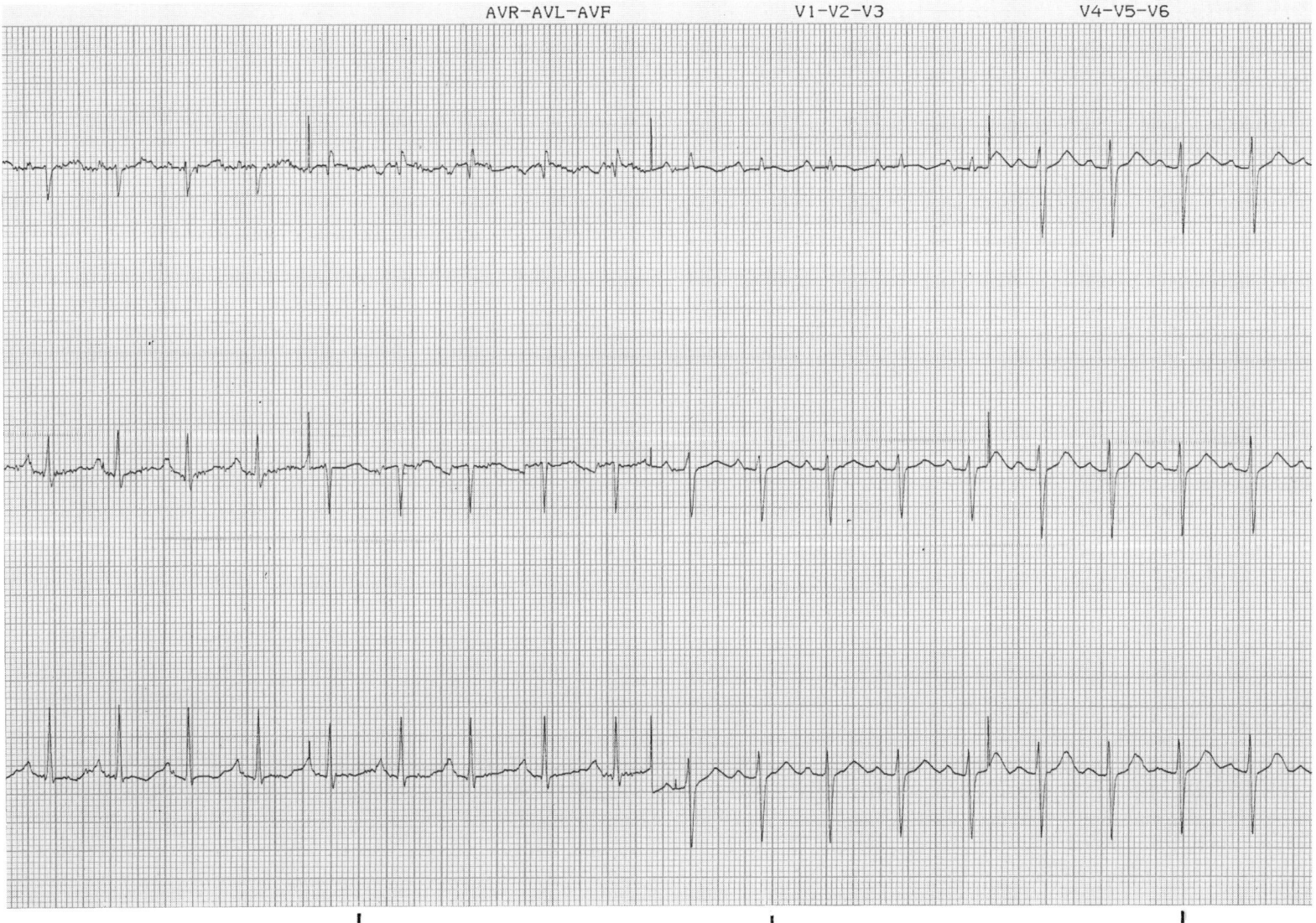

CASE 28

Rate and Rhythm

There is a P wave preceding each QRS complex, and the rhythm is normal sinus rhythm.

The heart rate is about 65 beats per minute.

Intervals

PR interval: 0.28s
QRS duration: 0.06s
QT interval: 0.60s

The prolonged PR interval indicates a first-degree AV block. The prolonged QT interval is consistent with ischemia, electrolyte abnormality, or drug effect.

QRS Axis

The QRS complex is positive in lead I and positive in lead aVF, so the QRS axis is in the normal quadrant. The isoelectric lead is III, so the QRS axis is +30 degrees.

Evidence for Atrial Enlargement

There is no evidence for atrial enlargement.

Evidence for Ventricular Hypertrophy

LVH: The sum of the S wave in V1 (14 mm) and the R wave in V5 (23 mm) is 37 mm. Thus there is left ventricular hypertrophy by voltage criteria.
RVH: The QRS axis is in the normal quadrant. There is no evidence for right ventricular hypertrophy.

R-Wave Progression

The R waves grow from V1 to V5, and the QRS complex becomes positive between V3 and V4. Thus there is normal (good) R-wave progression.

Evidence of Ischemia or Infarction

Anterior leads: There are downsloping ST-segment depressions with biphasic T waves in V2 to V6 and I, consistent with anterolateral ischemia or subendocardial infarction.
Inferior leads: There are ST-segment depressions and biphasic T waves in II and aVF and inverted T waves in III. These changes are consistent with inferior ischemia or subendocardial infarction.
ST-T waves: The ST-T wave changes seen in the anterior and inferior leads are more than one would expect for secondary changes from left ventricular hypertrophy. Secondary changes would have been confined to the apical leads.

Summary

Normal sinus rhythm at 65 bpm, with first-degree AV block
Intervals: 0.28/0.06/0.60
QRS axis: +30 degrees
QT prolongation consistent with ischemia, electrolyte abnormality, or drug effect
Downsloping ST segments and biphasic T waves in V2 to V6 and I consistent with anterior ischemia or subendocardial infarction
Downsloping ST segments and biphasic T waves in II and aVF consistent with inferior ischemia or subendocardial infarction

CASE 28 □ 119

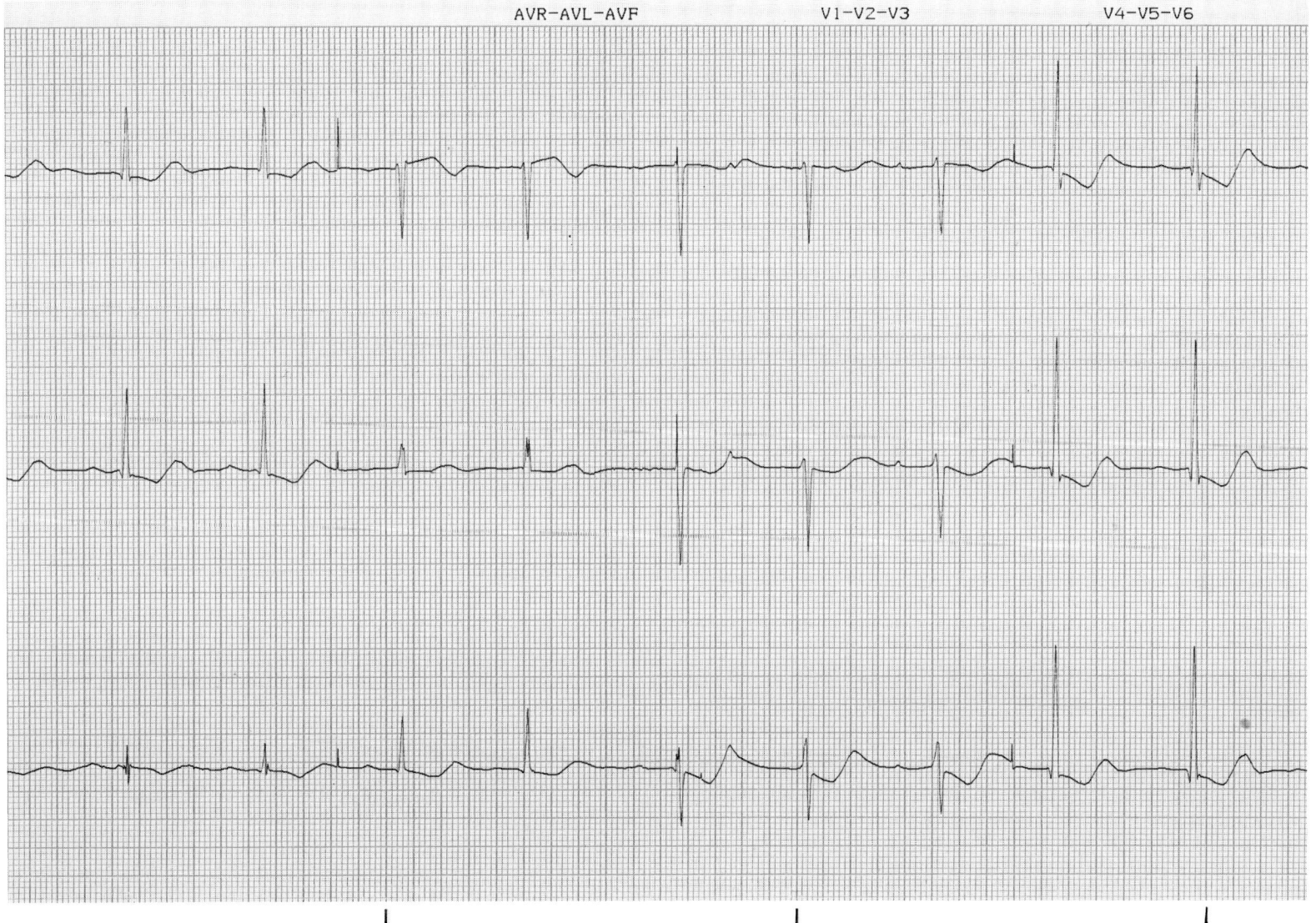

CASE 29

Rate and Rhythm

There is a P wave preceding each QRS complex, and the rhythm is probably normal sinus rhythm, although the P-wave shape in II, III, and aVF is not normal.

The heart rate is about 75 beats per minute.

Intervals

PR interval: 0.16s
QRS duration: 0.06s
QT interval: 0.36s

QRS Axis

The QRS complex is close to isoelectric in all the limb leads. Thus the QRS axis is indeterminate.

Evidence for Atrial Enlargement

There is no evidence for atrial enlargement.

Evidence for Ventricular Hypertrophy

LVH: The sum of the S wave in V1 (9 mm) and the R wave in V6 (1 mm) is 10 mm. There is no evidence of left ventricular hypertrophy by voltage criteria.

RVH: The QRS axis is indeterminate. There is no evidence for right ventricular hypertrophy.

R-Wave Progression

There are no R waves until V6; there are Q waves in V1 to V5. Thus there is poor R-wave progression.

Evidence of Ischemia or Infarction

Anterior leads: There are Q waves in V1 to V4, with ST-segment elevation in leads V1 to V6. These changes are consistent with an acute evolving anterior MI.

Inferior leads: The ST segments are downsloping, but they are not depressed. These changes are not specific.

Summary

Probable normal sinus rhythm at 75 bpm
Intervals: 0.16/0.06/0.36
QRS axis: indeterminate
Q waves in V1 to V4, with ST-segment elevation in leads V1 to V6, consistent with acute, evolving anterior MI

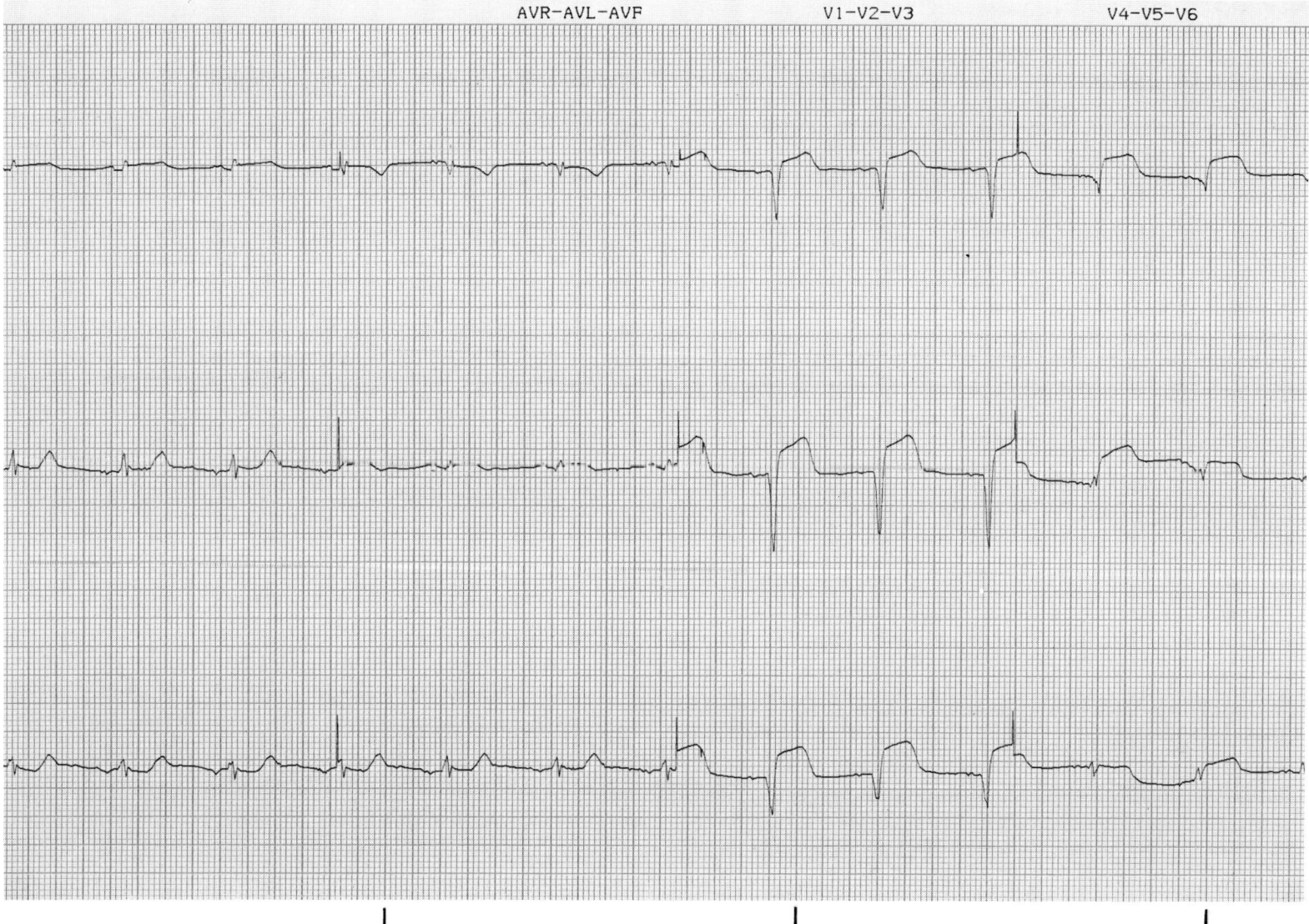

CASE 30

Rate and Rhythm

There is a P wave preceding each QRS complex, and the rhythm is normal sinus rhythm.

The heart rate is about 65 beats per minute.

Intervals

PR interval: 0.28s
QRS duration: 0.16s
QT interval: 0.40s

The prolonged PR interval indicates a first-degree AV block. The prolonged QRS duration indicates a bundle-branch block; examination of lead V1 shows an RSR' pattern, so this is a right bundle-branch block.

QRS Axis

The QRS complex is positive in lead I and negative in lead aVF, so the QRS axis is in the leftward quadrant. The isoelectric lead is II, so the QRS axis is −30 degrees. This is left axis deviation, consistent with left anterior hemiblock.

Evidence for Atrial Enlargement

There is no evidence for atrial enlargement.

Evidence for Ventricular Hypertrophy

LVH: The sum of the S wave in V1 (2 mm) and the R wave in V5 (13 mm) is 15 mm. There is no evidence of left ventricular hypertrophy by voltage criteria.
RVH: We cannot diagnose right ventricular hypertrophy in the setting of a right bundle-branch block.

R-Wave Progression

The R-wave progression appears to be normal.

Evidence of Ischemia or Infarction

Anterior leads: There is no specific evidence of ischemia or infarction.
Inferior leads: There is no specific evidence of ischemia or infarction.
ST-T waves: The ST-segment depressions in the anterior leads are secondary ST-T wave changes from the right bundle-branch block.

Summary

Normal sinus rhythm at 65 bpm, with first-degree AV block
Intervals: 0.28/0.16/0.40
QRS axis: −30 degrees
Right bundle-branch block with left anterior hemiblock

CASE 30

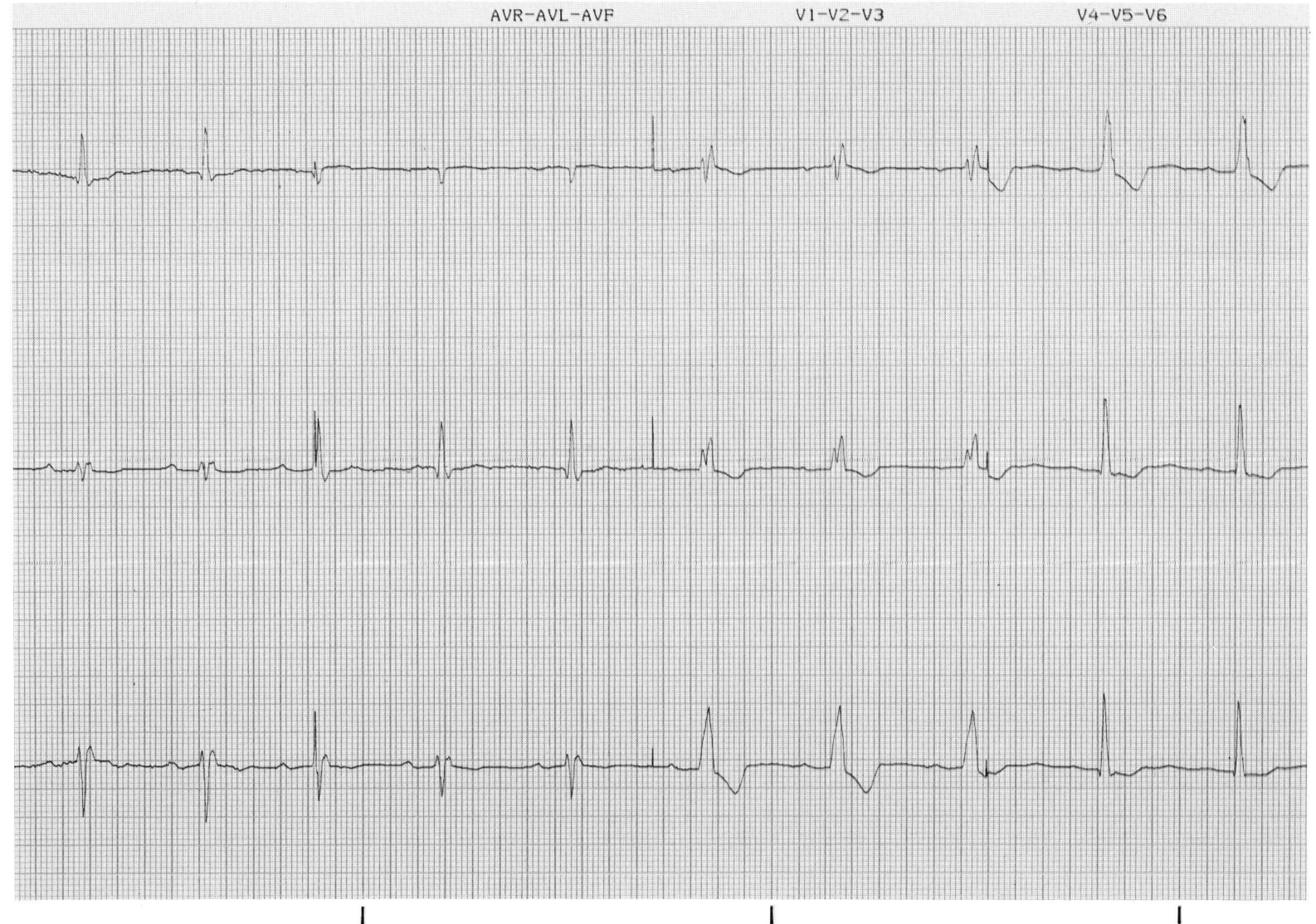

CASE 31

Rate and Rhythm

There is a P wave preceding each QRS complex, and the rhythm is normal sinus rhythm.

The heart rate is about 80 beats per minute.

Intervals

PR interval: 0.10s
QRS duration: 0.08s
QT interval: 0.36s

The short PR interval and the slurred upstrokes of the QRS complexes indicate that there is preexcitation. This is a tracing from a patient with Wolff-Parkinson-White syndrome.

QRS Axis

The QRS complex is positive in lead I and positive in lead aVF, so the QRS axis is in the normal quadrant. Lead aVL is closest to being isoelectric, but it is slightly negative. The QRS axis is thus between +60 and +90 degrees, or about +75 degrees.

Evidence for Atrial Enlargement

There is no evidence for atrial enlargement.

Evidence for Ventricular Hypertrophy

LVH: The sum of the S wave in V1 (1 mm) and the R wave in V5 (22 mm) is 23 mm. There is no evidence of left ventricular hypertrophy by voltage criteria.

RVH: The QRS axis is in the normal quadrant. There is no evidence for right ventricular hypertrophy.

R-Wave Progression

The R waves are tall in V1, and they grow from V1 to V5. The reasons for tall R waves in V1 include counterclockwise rotation, faulty lead placement, and Wolff-Parkinson-White syndrome. We know there is not a right bundle-branch block, and in the absence of inferior ischemic changes, tall R waves in V1 are unlikely to be due to posterior MI.

Evidence of Ischemia or Infarction

Anterior leads: There are downsloping ST-segment depressions in V1 to V5. There is a Q wave in aVL.
Inferior leads: There are downsloping ST-segment depressions in II, III, and aVF.
ST-T waves: While these changes are of concern in anterolateral and inferior ischemia or subendocardial infarction, in this 24-year-old patient with Wolff-Parkinson-White syndrome it is likely that these are repolarization changes.

Summary

Normal sinus rhythm at 80 bpm
Intervals: 0.10/0.08/0.36
QRS axis: +75 degrees
Wolff-Parkinson-White syndrome, with delta waves indicating preexcitation
Diffuse ST-segment depressions probably due to repolarization abnormalities from Wolff-Parkinson-White syndrome

CASE 31 • 125

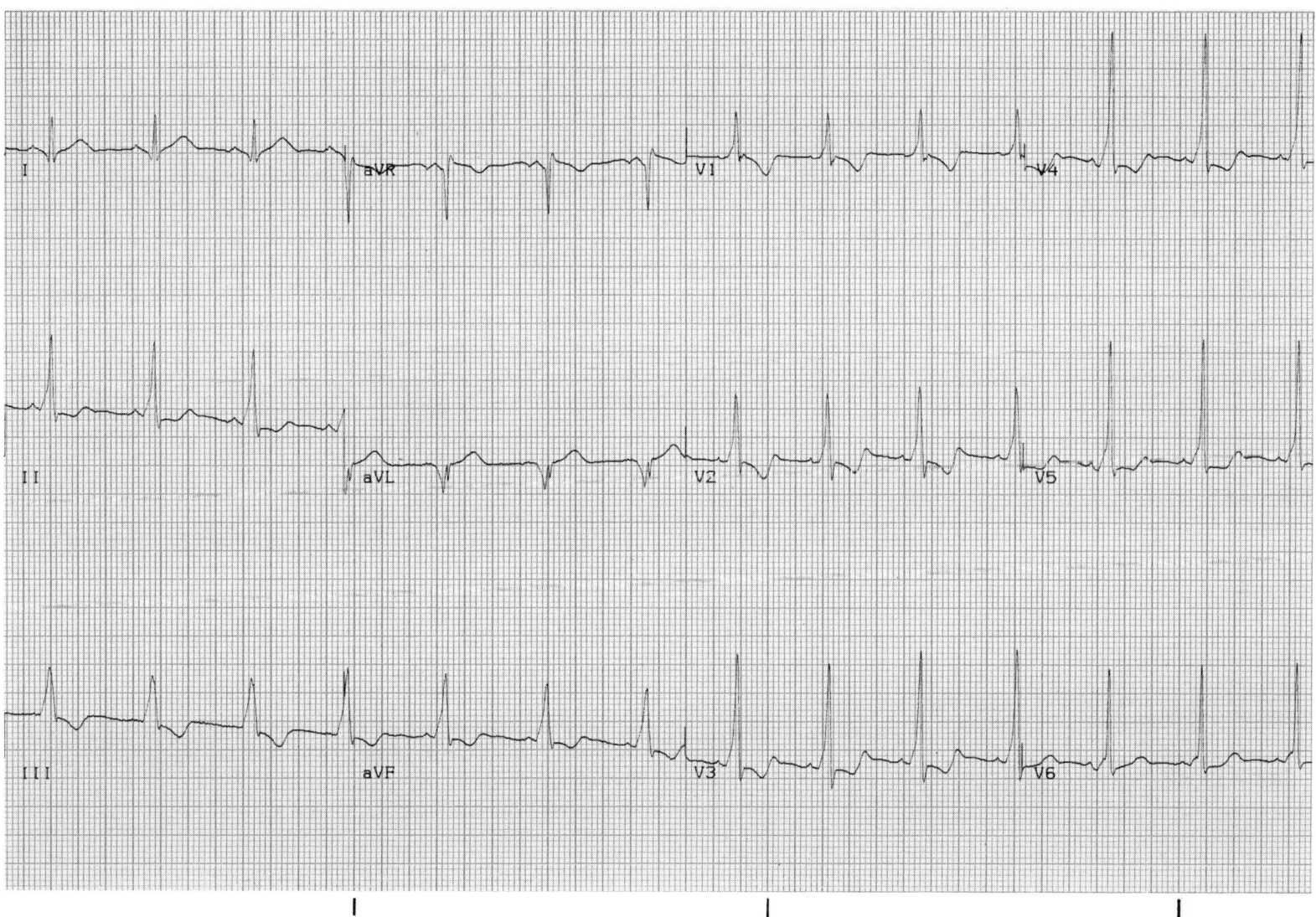

CASE 32

Rate and Rhythm

There are no visible P waves, and the rhythm is irregular. The QRS complexes are narrow, so this is a supraventricular rhythm. This is atrial fibrillation.

The heart rate varies throughout the tracing. Using the 6-s method, there are 8 QRS complexes in 6 s, so the average rate is about 80 beats per minute. Thus this is atrial fibrillation with moderate ventricular response.

Intervals

PR interval: not applicable (n.a.)
QRS duration: 0.06s
QT interval: 0.36s

QRS Axis

The QRS complex is positive in lead I and positive in lead aVF, so the QRS axis is in the normal quadrant. Lead aVL is closest to isoelectric lead, so the QRS axis is close to +60 degrees. Since the QRS complex in aVL is slightly negative, the QRS axis is slightly greater than +60 degrees, about +70 degrees.

Evidence for Atrial Enlargement

Since there are no P waves, we cannot assess for atrial enlargement.

Evidence for Ventricular Hypertrophy

LVH: The sum of the S wave in V1 (7 mm) and the R wave in V5 (18 mm) is 25 mm. There is no evidence of left ventricular hypertrophy by voltage criteria.

RVH: The QRS axis is in the normal quadrant. There is no evidence for right ventricular hypertrophy.

R-Wave Progression

The R waves grow from V1 to V6, and the QRS complexes become mostly positive around V4 to V5. This is normal R-wave progression.

Evidence of Ischemia or Infarction

Anterior leads: There are T-wave inversions in leads V2 to V6, with ST-segment depression in V5 and V6. While changes confined to V5 and V6 might be digoxin effect, the changes from V2 to V6 suggest anterior ischemia or subendocardial infarction.

Inferior leads: The T waves are flat, and there are nonspecific ST-T wave abnormalities in the inferior leads.

Summary

Atrial fibrillation with moderate ventricular response
Intervals: n.a./0.06/0.36
QRS axis: +70 degrees
T-wave inversions in V2 to V6 with ST-segment depression in V6 consistent with anterior ischemia or subendocardial infarction

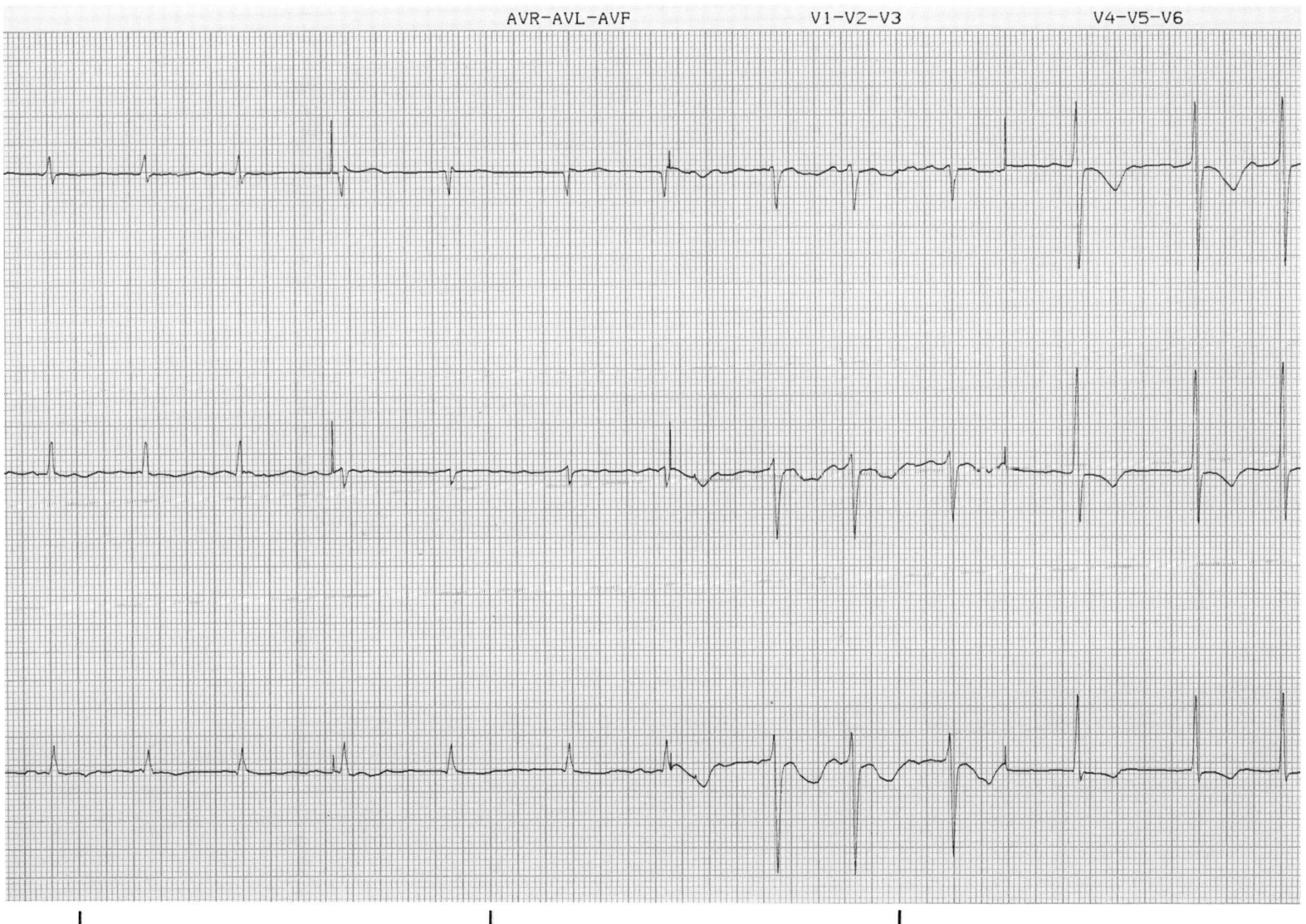

CASE 33

Rate and Rhythm

There are P waves in this rhythm, but they are closer to the preceding QRS complex than to the next one. There is still one P wave for each QRS complex. Examination of lead II reveals that the P waves are negative and occur in the middle of the upright T waves. This is an example of accelerated junctional tachycardia with retrograde P waves.

The heart rate is about 135 beats per minute.

Intervals

PR interval: not applicable
QRS duration: 0.06s
QT interval: 0.32s

QRS Axis

The QRS complex is positive in lead I and positive in lead aVF, so the QRS axis is in the normal quadrant. The isoelectric lead is closest to III and aVL, so the QRS axis is between +60 and +30 degrees, or about +45 degrees.

Evidence for Atrial Enlargement

The P waves do not originate from the sinus, so we cannot assess for atrial enlargement.

Evidence for Ventricular Hypertrophy

LVH: The sum of the S wave in V1 (14 mm) and the R wave in V5 (15 mm) is 29 mm. There is no evidence of left ventricular hypertrophy by voltage criteria.
RVH: The QRS axis is in the normal quadrant. There is no evidence for right ventricular hypertrophy.

R-Wave Progression

The R waves grow from V1 to V5, and the QRS complex becomes mostly positive between V4 and V5. The R-wave progression is normal.

Evidence of Ischemia or Infarction

The retrograde P waves occur in the middle of the T waves, which gives the impression of T-wave inversion. There are no specific changes of ischemia or infarction. There are nonspecific ST-T wave abnormalities.

Summary

Junctional tachycardia at 135 bpm, with retrograde P waves
Intervals: n.a./0.06/0.32
QRS axis: +45 degrees
Nonspecific ST-T wave abnormalities
Junctional tachycardia raises the possibility of digoxin toxicity.

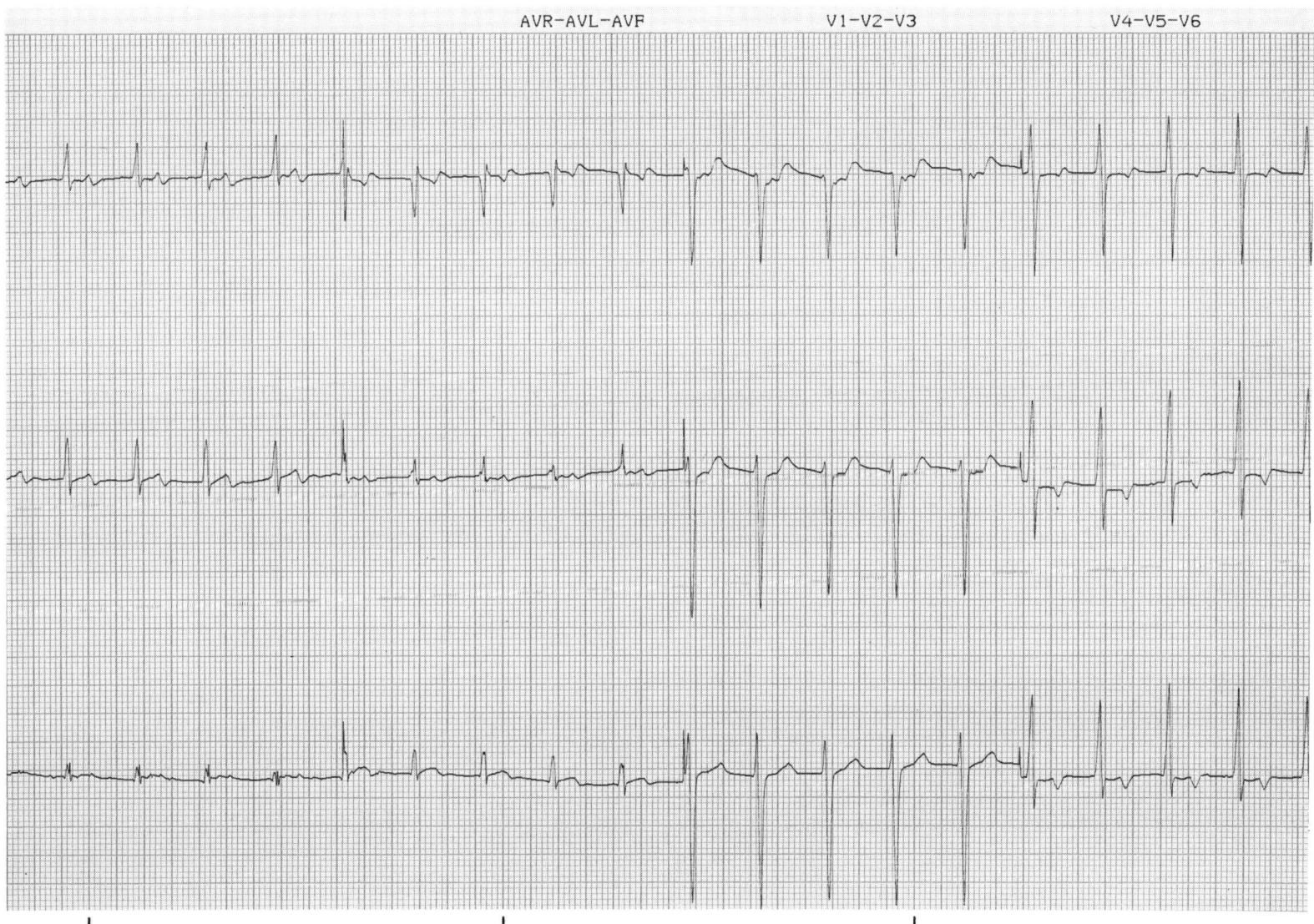

CASE 34

Rate and Rhythm

The P waves are difficult to see, but there is a P wave preceding each QRS complex, and the rhythm is normal sinus rhythm.

The heart rate is about 75 beats per minute.

Intervals

PR interval: 0.16s
QRS duration: 0.08s
QT interval.   0.40s

QRS Axis

The QRS complex is positive in lead I and negative in lead aVF, so the QRS axis is in the leftward quadrant. Leads II and aVF are closest to isoelectric, so the QRS axis is between 0 and −30 degrees, or about −15 degrees. This is leftward axis.

Evidence for Atrial Enlargement

There is no evidence for atrial enlargement.

Evidence for Ventricular Hypertrophy

LVH: The sum of the S wave in V1 (11 mm) and the R wave in V5 (9 mm) is 20 mm. There is no evidence of left ventricular hypertrophy by voltage criteria.

RVH: The QRS axis is in the leftward quadrant. There is no evidence for right ventricular hypertrophy.

R-Wave Progression

There are Q waves in V1 to V3. Thus there is poor R-wave progression.

Evidence of Ischemia or Infarction

Anterior leads: There are Q waves in V1 to V3, consistent with an anterior MI.
Inferior leads: There are no specific changes consistent with ischemia.
ST-T waves: There are nonspecific ST-T wave abnormalities.

Summary

Normal sinus rhythm at 75 bpm, with baseline artifact
Intervals: 0.16/0.08/0.40
QRS axis: −15 degrees
Leftward axis
Q waves in leads V1 to V3 consistent with anterior MI
Nonspecific ST-T wave abnormalities

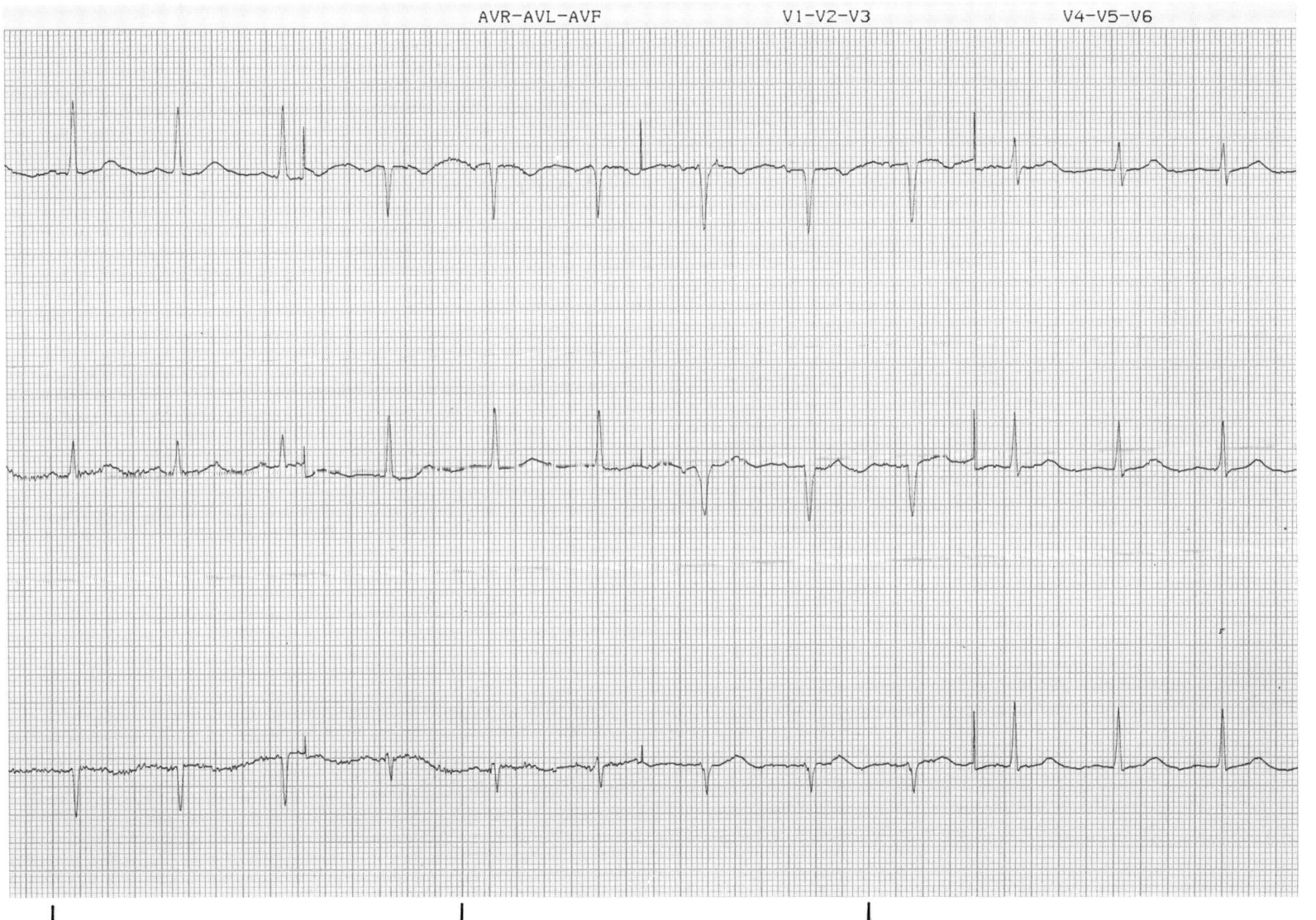

CASE 35

Rate and Rhythm

There is a P wave preceding each QRS complex, and the rhythm is sinus tachycardia.

The heart rate is about 105 beats per minute.

Intervals

PR interval: 0.14s
QRS duration: 0.06s
QT interval: 0.36s

QRS Axis

The QRS complex is positive in lead I and positive in lead aVF, so the QRS axis is in the normal quadrant. The isoelectric lead is aVL, so the QRS axis is +60 degrees.

Evidence for Atrial Enlargement

There is no evidence for atrial enlargement.

Evidence for Ventricular Hypertrophy

LVH: The sum of the S wave in V1 (10 mm) and the R wave in V5 (15 mm) is 25 mm. There is no evidence of left ventricular hypertrophy by voltage criteria.

RVH: The QRS axis is in the normal quadrant. There is no evidence for right ventricular hypertrophy.

R-Wave Progression

The R waves grow slowly from V1 to V3, but the QRS complex becomes positive between V4 and V5. The R-wave progression is close to normal.

Evidence of Ischemia or Infarction

Anterior leads: There are T-wave inversions in V2 to V5 with downsloping ST-segment depression in V4 to V6, consistent with anteroapical ischemia or subendocardial infarction.
Inferior leads: There are nonspecific ST-T wave abnormalities.

Summary

Sinus tachycardia at 105 bpm
Intervals: 0.14/0.06/0.36
QRS axis: +60 degrees
T-wave inversions in leads V2 to V5 with downsloping ST-segment depression in V4 to V6 consistent with anteroapical ischemia or subendocardial infarction

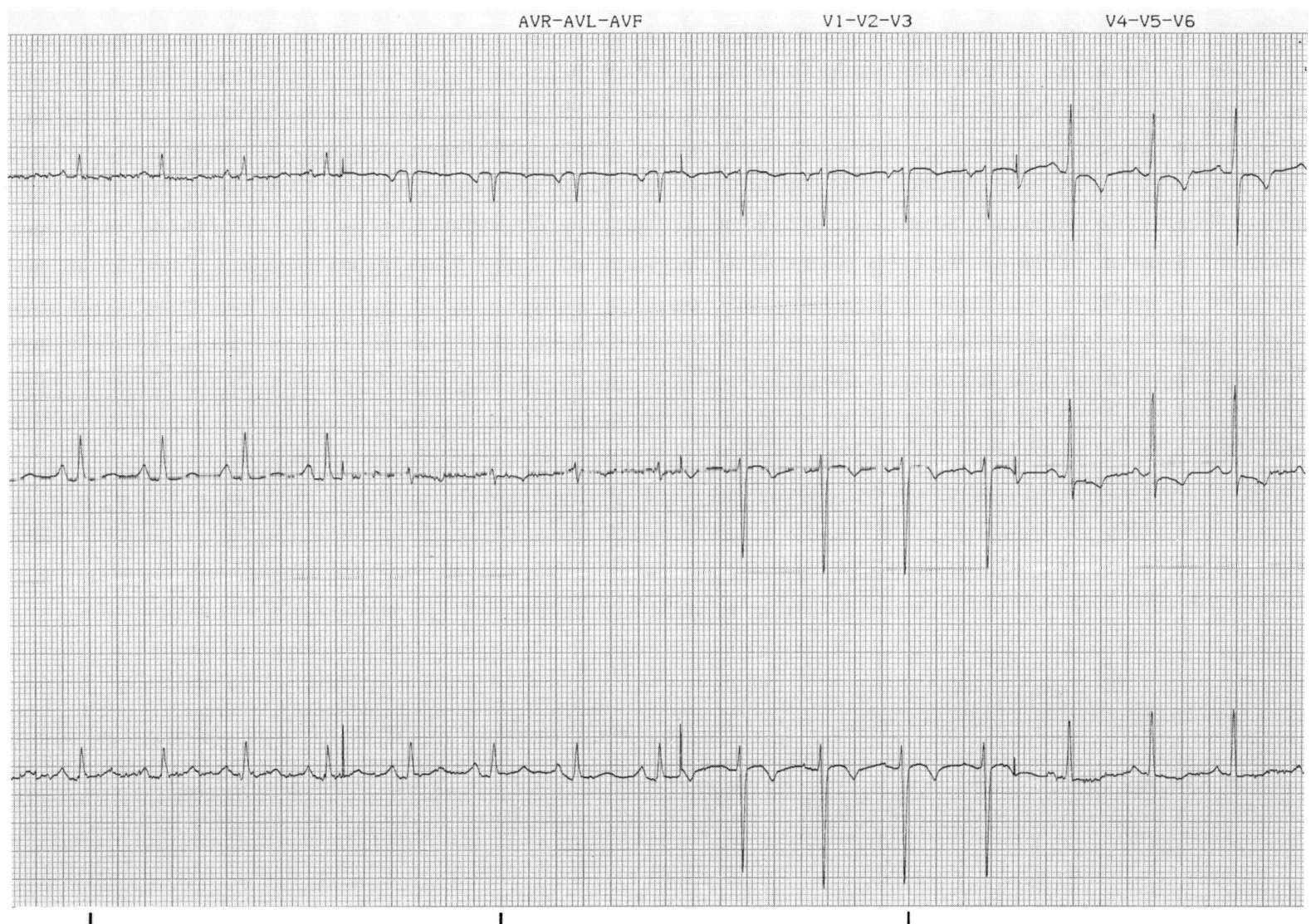

CASE 36

Rate and Rhythm

There is a P wave preceding each QRS complex, and the rhythm is sinus tachycardia.

The heart rate is just over 100 beats per minute.

Intervals

PR interval: 0.20s
QRS duration: 0.12s
QT interval: 0.36s

The wide QRS complex indicates that there is a bundle-branch block. Examination of the QRS complex in V1 shows a predominantly positive QRS complex. It is not the RSR' typical of right bundle-branch block, but V2 and V3 show some splintering of the QRS complex. This is an atypical right bundle-branch block.

QRS Axis

The QRS complex is isoelectric in lead I and negative in lead aVF, so the QRS axis is in the leftward quadrant. The isoelectric lead is I, so the QRS axis is −90 degrees. This is left axis deviation.

Evidence for Atrial Enlargement

In lead II, the P wave is both tall and wide, meeting criteria for both left and right atrial enlargement. In lead V1, the terminal phase of the biphasic P wave is greater than 1 mm, consistent with left atrial enlargement. Thus we may call the condition biatrial enlargement.

Evidence for Ventricular Hypertrophy

We cannot see the R waves clearly, but there does not appear to be evidence of left or right ventricular hypertrophy.

R-Wave Progression

The R waves appear to start out tall in V1. This may be due to posterior MI or right bundle-branch block. The R waves in V4 to V6 are not as tall as in V1 to V3, so this is not simply counterclockwise rotation.

Evidence of Ischemia or Infarction

Anterior leads: The ST and T waves are difficult to interpret with the right bundle-branch block but do not appear to be specific for ischemia.

Inferior leads: There are Q waves in II, III, and aVF, as well as tall R waves in V1 and V2, consistent with an inferoposterior MI.

Summary

Sinus tachycardia at 105 bpm
Intervals: 0.20/0.12/0.36
QRS axis: −90 degrees
Right bundle-branch block with left anterior hemiblock
Biatrial enlargement
Q waves in II, III, and aVF with tall R waves in V1 and V2 consistent with inferoposterior MI

CASE 36 □ 135

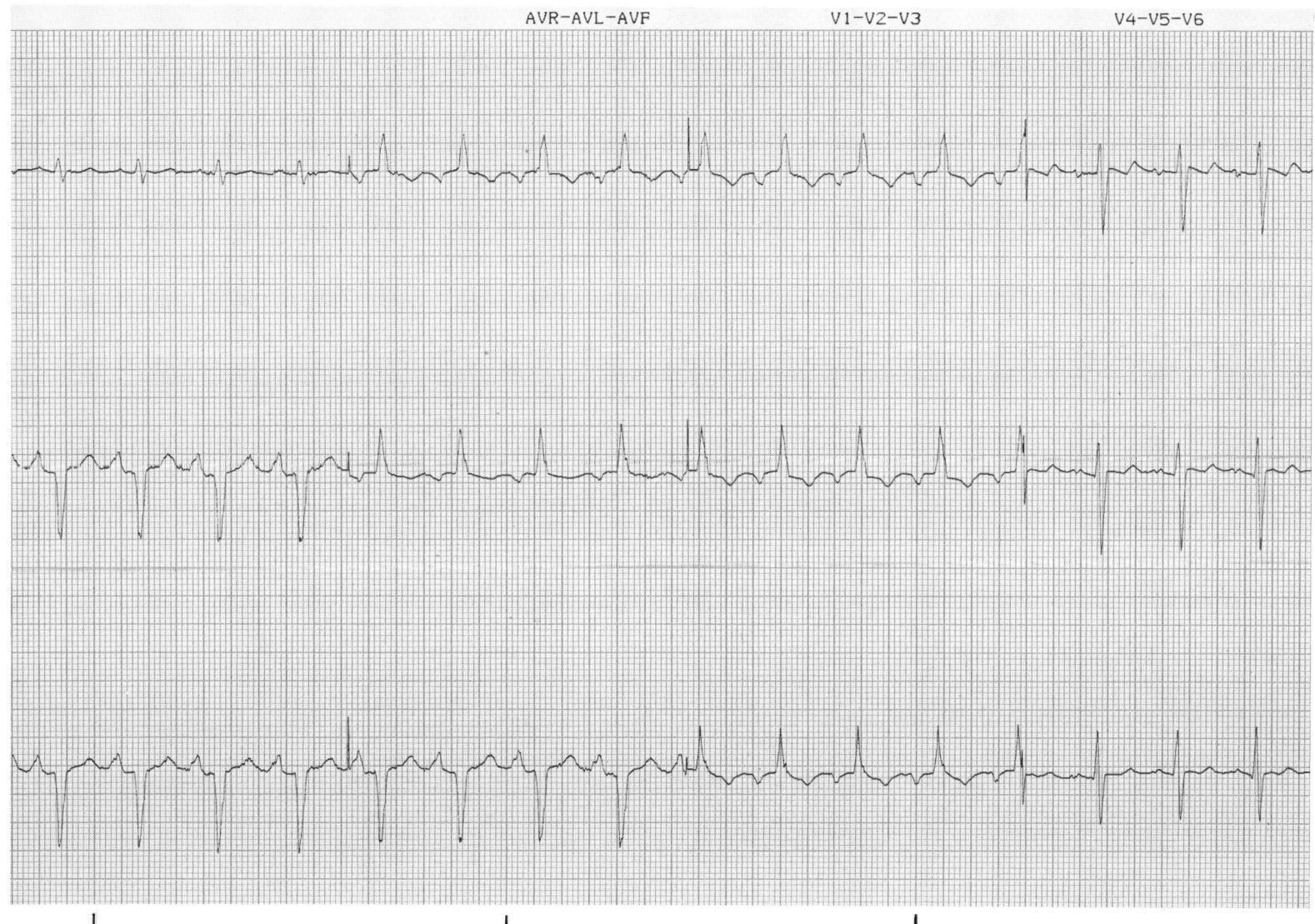

CASE 37

Rate and Rhythm

There is a P wave preceding each QRS complex, and the rhythm is normal sinus rhythm.

The heart rate is about 85 beats per minute.

Intervals

PR interval: 0.18s
QRS duration: 0.06s
QT interval: 0.40s

QRS Axis

The QRS complex is negative in lead I and positive in lead aVF, so the QRS axis is in the rightward quadrant. The isoelectric lead is aVR, so the QRS axis is +120 degrees. Right axis deviation should make us consider right ventricular hypertrophy.

Evidence for Atrial Enlargement

In lead II, the P waves are notched and wider than 2.5 mm. In lead V1, the P waves are biphasic, and the terminal part is wider than 1 mm. Thus there is left atrial enlargement.

Evidence for Ventricular Hypertrophy

LVH: The sum of the S wave in V1 (0 mm) and the R wave in V6 (1 mm) is 1 mm. There is no evidence of left ventricular hypertrophy by voltage criteria.

RVH: There is right axis deviation to +120 degrees, meeting the axis criteria for right ventricular hypertrophy. Examination of V1 shows an R/S ratio greater than 1 (and examination of V6 shows an R/S ratio less than 1), so the voltage criteria are satisfied. There is right ventricular hypertrophy.

R-Wave Progression

There are Q waves in V1 to V5, so there is poor R-wave progression.

Evidence of Ischemia or Infarction

Anterior leads: There are Q waves in V1 to V5, I, and aVL consistent with an anterolateral MI. The ST segments are slightly elevated in V1 and V2, suggesting that the MI might be acute.

Inferior leads: There are no specific changes of ischemia or infarction.

Summary

Normal sinus rhythm at 85 bpm
Intervals: 0.18/0.06/0.40
QRS axis: +120 degrees
Left atrial enlargement
Right ventricular hypertrophy
Q waves in V1 to V5, I, and aVL consistent with anterolateral MI, possibly acute

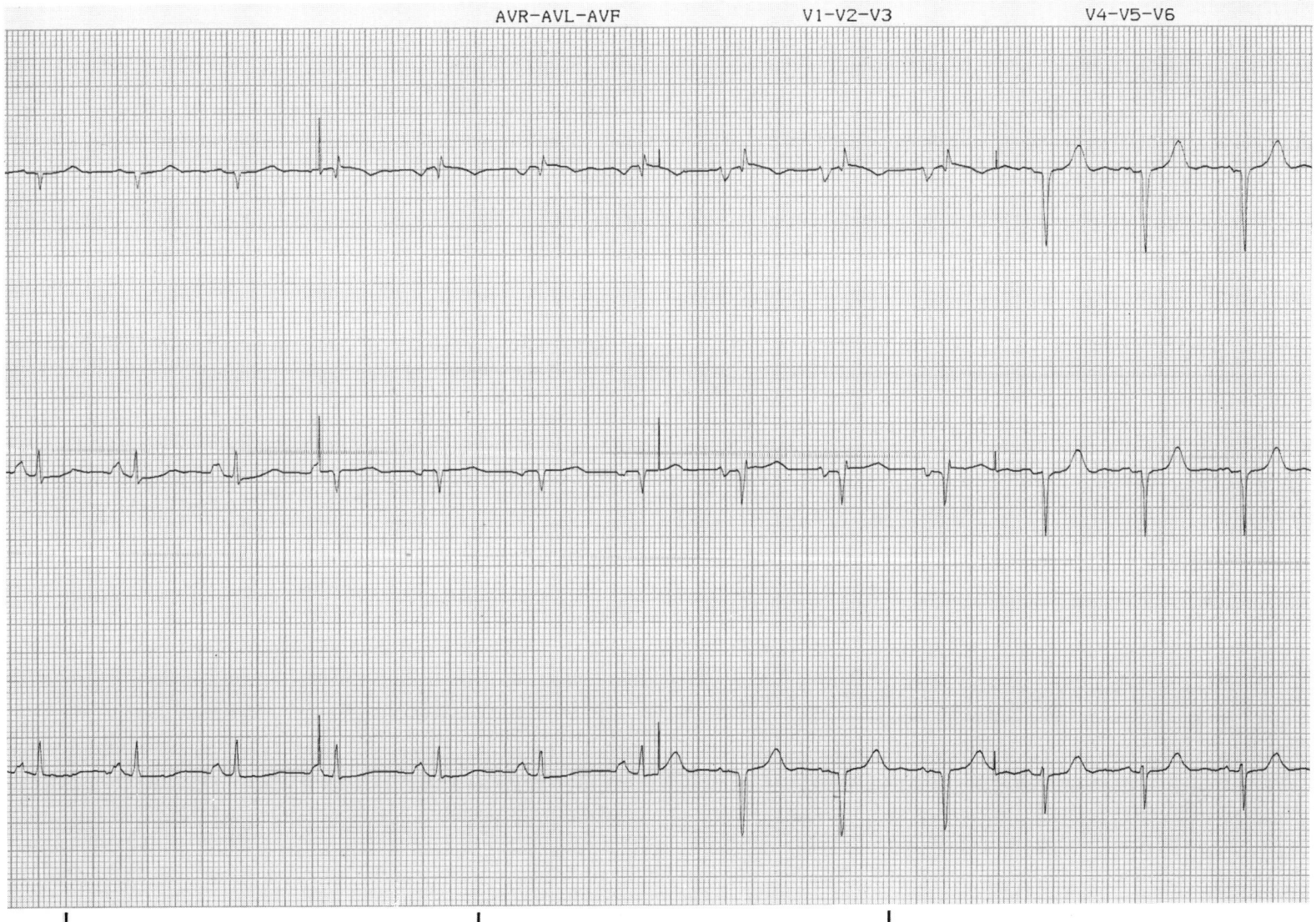

CASE 38

Rate and Rhythm

There is a P wave preceding each QRS complex, and the rhythm is normal sinus rhythm.

The heart rate is about 80 beats per minute.

Intervals

PR interval: 0.16s
QRS duration: 0.16s
QT interval: 0.40s

The prolonged QRS duration indicates a bundle-branch block. Examination of lead V1 shows a positive QRS, and lead V2 shows the typical RSR′ of right bundle-branch block.

QRS Axis

The QRS complex is positive in lead I and isoelectric in lead aVF, so the QRS axis is about zero.

Evidence for Atrial Enlargement

In lead II, the P waves are notched and widened to more than 2.5 mm. In lead V1, the P waves are biphasic, with the terminal part wider than 1 mm. Thus there is left atrial enlargement.

Evidence for Ventricular Hypertrophy

LVH: There is no evidence of left ventricular hypertrophy by voltage criteria.

RVH: We cannot assess for evidence of right ventricular hypertrophy with right bundle-branch block.

R-Wave Progression

The R waves of the RSR′ complex start out tall even in V1 and V2. These tall R waves may be due to posterior MI, counterclockwise rotation, or faulty lead placement.

Evidence of Ischemia or Infarction

Anterior leads: There is no specific evidence of ischemia or infarction.
Inferior leads: There are Q waves in III and aVF consistent with inferior MI. In this setting, the tall R waves in V1 and V2 are likely to indicate posterior involvement.
ST-T waves: There are changes secondary to the right bundle-branch block.

Summary

Normal sinus rhythm at 80 bpm
Intervals: 0.16/0.16/0.40
QRS axis: 0 degrees
Left atrial enlargement
Right bundle-branch block
Q waves in III and aVF with tall R waves in V1 and V2 consistent with inferoposterior MI

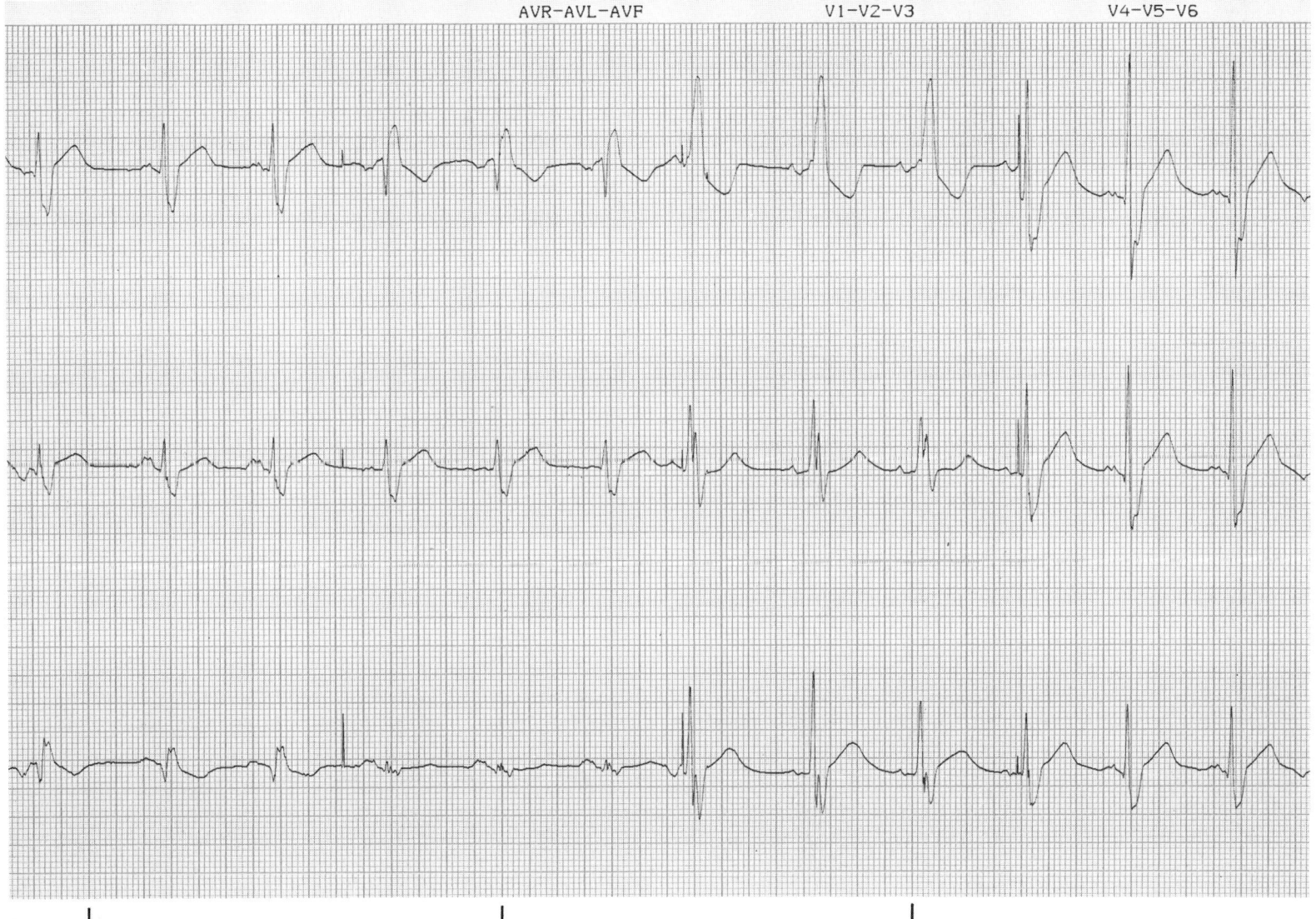

CASE 39

Rate and Rhythm

There is a P wave preceding each QRS complex, but closer examination reveals that the P waves in II, III, and aVF are inverted. Thus this is not sinus rhythm but an ectopic atrial rhythm from a low atrial pacemaker.

The heart rate is about 110 beats per minute.

Intervals

PR interval: not applicable (n.a.)
QRS duration: 0.06s
QT interval: 0.32s

QRS Axis

The QRS complex is isoelectric in lead I and positive in lead aVF, so the QRS axis is about +90 degrees.

Evidence for Atrial Enlargement

Because the rhythm is not sinus, we cannot assess for evidence of atrial enlargement.

Evidence for Ventricular Hypertrophy

LVH: The sum of the S wave in V1 (12 mm) and the R wave in V5 (3 mm) is 15 mm. There is no evidence of left ventricular hypertrophy by voltage criteria.

RVH: The QRS axis is +90 degrees on the border of right axis deviation. It does not meet the axis criteria for right ventricular hypertrophy. The QRS complex does show an R/S ratio of less than 1 in V6, so the tracing does meet the voltage criteria.

R-Wave Progression

The R waves grow slowly, and the QRS complex does not become positive even at V6. Thus there is poor R-wave progression.

Evidence of Ischemia or Infarction

Anterior leads: There is poor R-wave progression consistent with anterior MI.
Inferior leads: There are nonspecific ST-T wave abnormalities.

Summary

Ectopic atrial tachycardia at 110 bpm
Intervals: n.a./0.06/0.32
QRS axis: +90 degrees
Poor R-wave progression consistent with anterior MI
Nonspecific ST-T wave abnormalities

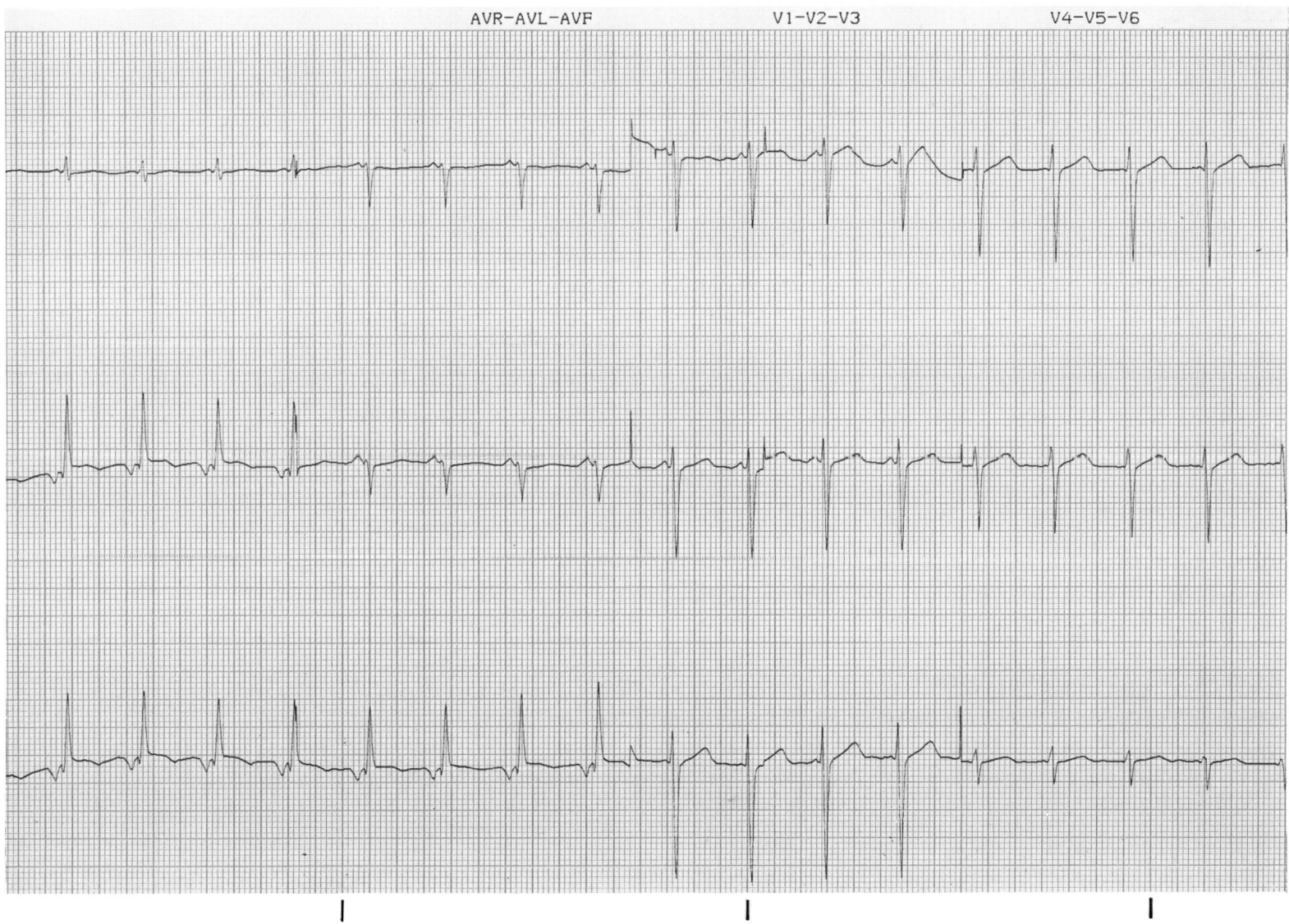

CASE 40

Rate and Rhythm

There are no visible P waves, and the rhythm is irregular. The QRS complexes are narrow for the most part, so the rhythm is supraventricular. This is atrial fibrillation.

There are two wide QRS complexes—the 6th beat and the 10th beat. While these may be premature ventricular contractions, they might also be aberrantly conducted beats. Examination of the rhythm shows that they occur after a long-short interval.

The overall ventricular rate is about 60 beats per minute, so this is atrial fibrillation with slow ventricular response.

Intervals

PR interval: not applicable (n.a.)
QRS duration: 0.08s
QT interval: 0.40s

QRS Axis

The QRS complex looks isoelectric in many of the limb leads, so the QRS axis is indeterminate.

Evidence for Atrial Enlargement

There are no P waves, so we cannot assess for atrial enlargement.

Evidence for Ventricular Hypertrophy

LVH: The sum of the S wave in V1 (3 mm) and the R wave in V5 (25 mm) is 28 mm. This does not meet criteria for left ventricular hypertrophy.
RVH: There is no evidence for right ventricular hypertrophy.

R-Wave Progression

The R waves grow and the QRS complexes become mostly positive around V3. The R-wave progression appears normal.

Evidence of Ischemia or Infarction

Anterior leads: There are upsloping ST-segment depressions in V2 to V4 that are nonspecific for ischemia or infarction.
Inferior leads: There are downsloping ST segments in II, III, and aVF that may suggest ischemia, but they too are nonspecific for ischemia or infarction.

Summary

Atrial fibrillation with slow ventricular response, with two aberrantly conducted beats
Intervals: n.a./0.08/0.40
QRS axis: indeterminate
Nonspecific ST-T wave abnormalities

CASE 40

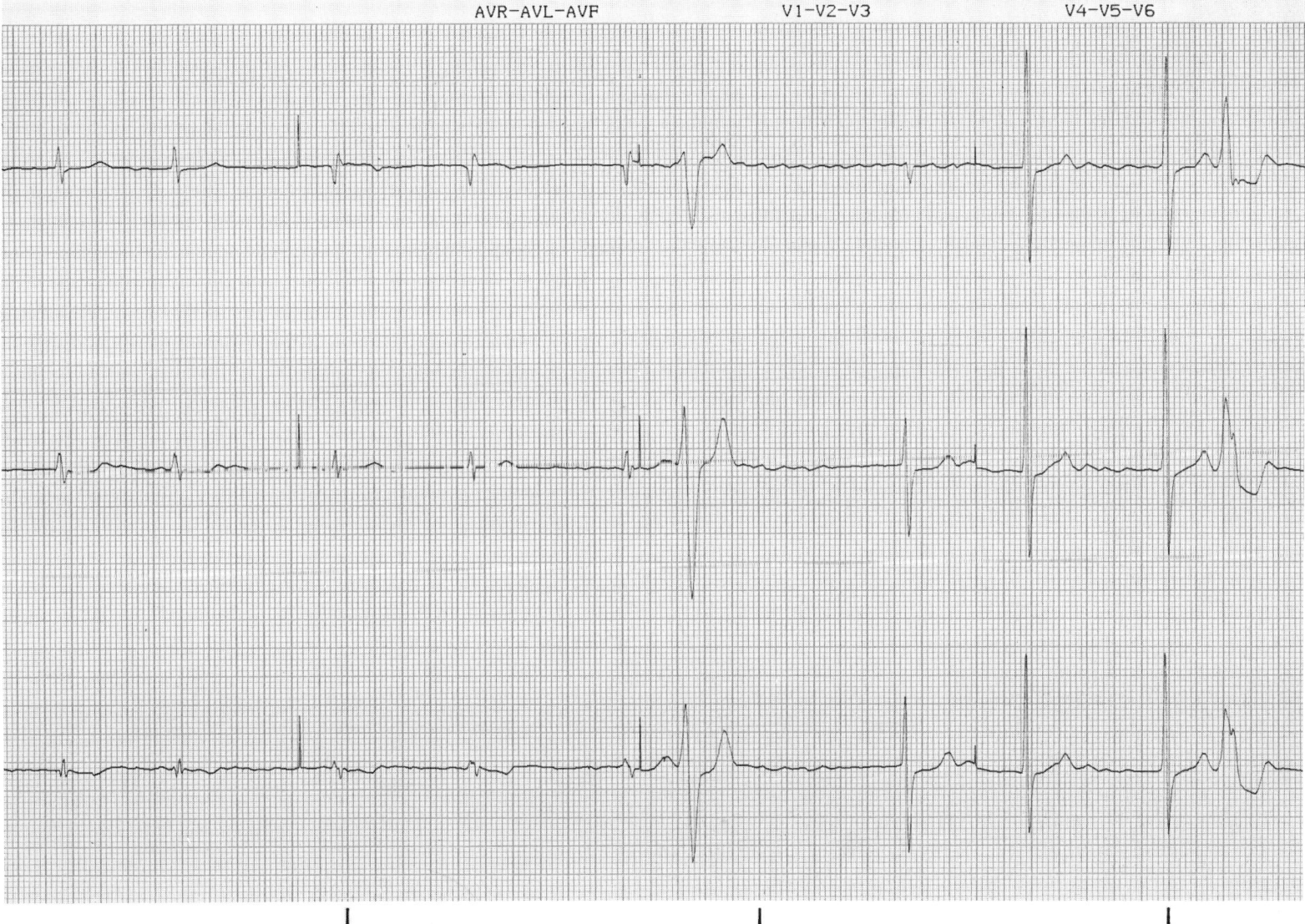

CASE 41

Rate and Rhythm

There are no clearly visible P waves, and the rhythm is irregular. The QRS complexes are narrow, so the rhythm is supraventricular. This is atrial fibrillation.

The heart rate is about 80 beats per minute, so this is atrial fibrillation with moderate ventricular response. The undulations seen in lead V1 may appear to be atrial flutter, but they are not regular.

Intervals

PR interval: not applicable (n.a.)
QRS duration: 0.10s
QT interval: 0.36s

The QRS duration is prolonged, so there is an interventricular conduction delay. It does not appear to be either left or right bundle-branch block type.

QRS Axis

The QRS complex is isoelectric in lead I and positive in lead aVF, so the QRS axis is +90 degrees.

Evidence for Atrial Enlargement

There are no P waves, so we cannot assess for atrial enlargement.

Evidence for Ventricular Hypertrophy

LVH: The sum of the S wave in V1 (11 mm) and the R wave in V5 (2 mm) is 13 mm. There is no evidence of left ventricular hypertrophy by voltage criteria.
RVH: There is no evidence for right ventricular hypertrophy.

R-Wave Progression

The R waves do not grow very much, and the QRS complex stays mostly negative. Thus there is poor R-wave progression.

Evidence of Ischemia or Infarction

Anterior leads: There is poor R-wave progression consistent with anterior MI. There are biphasic to inverted T waves in V4 to V6 consistent with apical ischemia or subendocardial infarction.
Inferior leads: There are nonspecific ST-T wave abnormalities.

Summary

Atrial fibrillation with moderate ventricular response
Intervals: n.a./0.10/0.36
QRS axis: +90 degrees
Interventricular conduction delay
Poor R-wave progression consistent with anterior MI
Biphasic to inverted T waves in V4 to V6 consistent with apical ischemia or subendocardial infarction

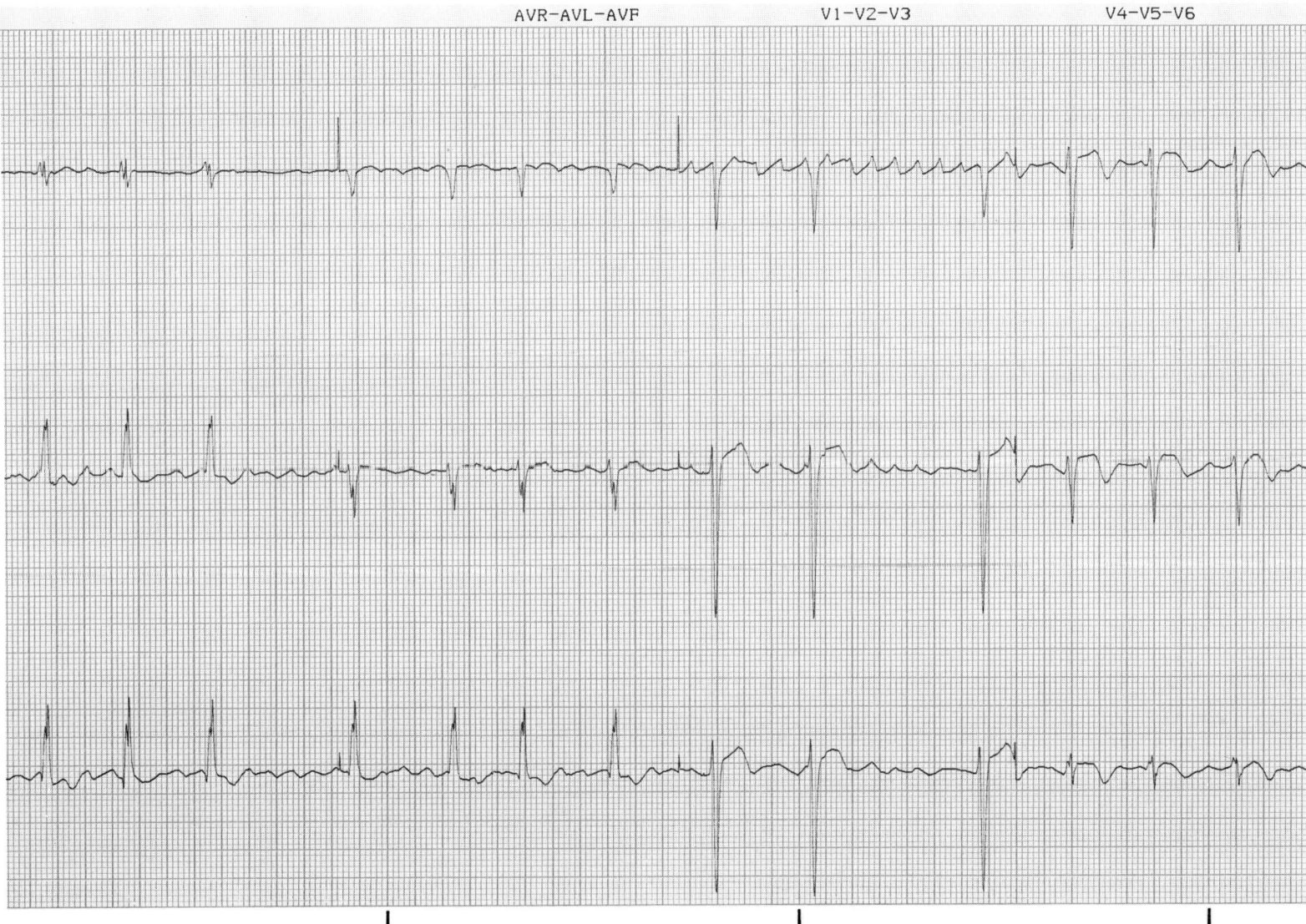

CASE 42

Rate and Rhythm

There is a P wave preceding each QRS complex, and the rhythm is normal sinus rhythm.

The heart rate is 80 beats per minute.

Intervals

PR interval: 0.12s
QRS duration: 0.06s
QT interval: 0.36s

QRS Axis

The QRS complex is positive in lead I and negative in lead aVF, so the QRS axis is in the leftward quadrant. The isoelectric lead is II, so the QRS axis is −30 degrees. This is left axis deviation. In this tracing, this could be due to left ventricular hypertrophy or left anterior hemiblock.

Evidence for Atrial Enlargement

There is no evidence for atrial enlargement.

Evidence for Ventricular Hypertrophy

LVH: The sum of the S wave in V1 (15 mm) and the R wave in V5 (28 mm) is 43 mm. Thus there is left ventricular hypertrophy by voltage criteria. Note also that the R wave in aVL is over 11 mm, meeting another definition of left ventricular hypertrophy.

RVH: The QRS axis is in the leftward quadrant. There is no evidence for right ventricular hypertrophy.

R-Wave Progression

The R waves do not grow very much from V1 to V3, so there is poor R-wave progression.

Evidence of Ischemia or Infarction

Anterior leads: There is poor R-wave progression from V1 to V3, and there are ST-segment elevations in V2 to V6 consistent with acute evolving anterior MI.

Inferior leads: There are no specific changes consistent with ischemia.

Summary

Normal sinus rhythm at 80 bpm
Intervals: 0.12/0.06/0.36
QRS axis: −30 degrees
Left ventricular hypertrophy with left axis deviation
ST-segment elevations in V2 to V6 with poor R-wave progression consistent with acute evolving anterior MI

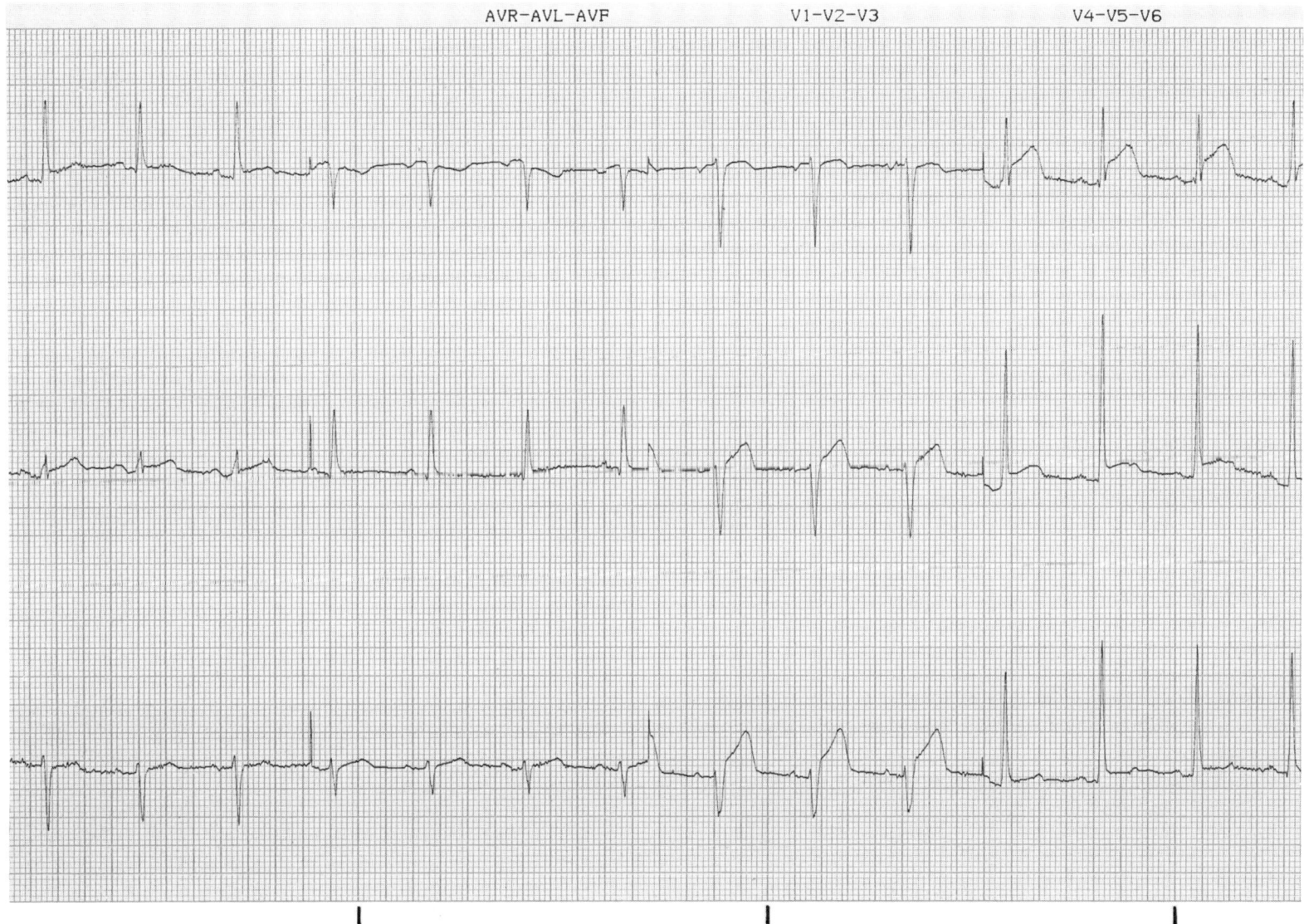

CASE 43

Rate and Rhythm

There is a P wave preceding each QRS complex, and the rhythm is sinus bradycardia.

The heart rate is about 45 beats per minute.

Intervals

PR interval: 0.20s
QRS duration: 0.06s
QT interval: 0.44s

QRS Axis

The QRS complex is positive in lead I and positive in lead aVF, so the QRS axis is in the normal quadrant. The isoelectric lead is III, so the QRS axis is +30 degrees.

Evidence for Atrial Enlargement

In lead II, the P waves are widened to 2.5 mm, suggestive of left atrial enlargement, but lead V1 does not show the expected changes.

Evidence for Ventricular Hypertrophy

LVH: The sum of the S wave in V1 (7 mm) and the R wave in V5 (11 mm) is 18 mm. There is no evidence of left ventricular hypertrophy by voltage criteria.

RVH: The QRS axis is in the normal quadrant. There is no evidence for right ventricular hypertrophy.

R-Wave Progression

The R waves do not grow very much from V1 to V3. Thus there is pooor R-wave progression.

Evidence of Ischemia or Infarction

Anterior leads: There is poor R-wave progression. There is ST-segment depression in V2 consistent with anteroseptal ischemia. There is ST-segment depression and T-wave inversion in I and aVL consistent with lateral ischemia.

Inferior leads: There is ST-segment elevation in II, III, and aVF consistent with acute inferior MI. In this setting, the ST-segment depressions in V2 may indicate posterior injury.

Summary

Sinus bradycardia at 45 bpm
Intervals: 0.20/0.06/0.44
QRS axis: +30 degrees
ST-segment elevation in II, III, and aVF consistent with acute inferior MI
ST-segment depression in V2 consistent with anteroseptal ischemia or posterior injury
ST-segment depression and T-wave inversion in I and aVL consistent with lateral ischemia

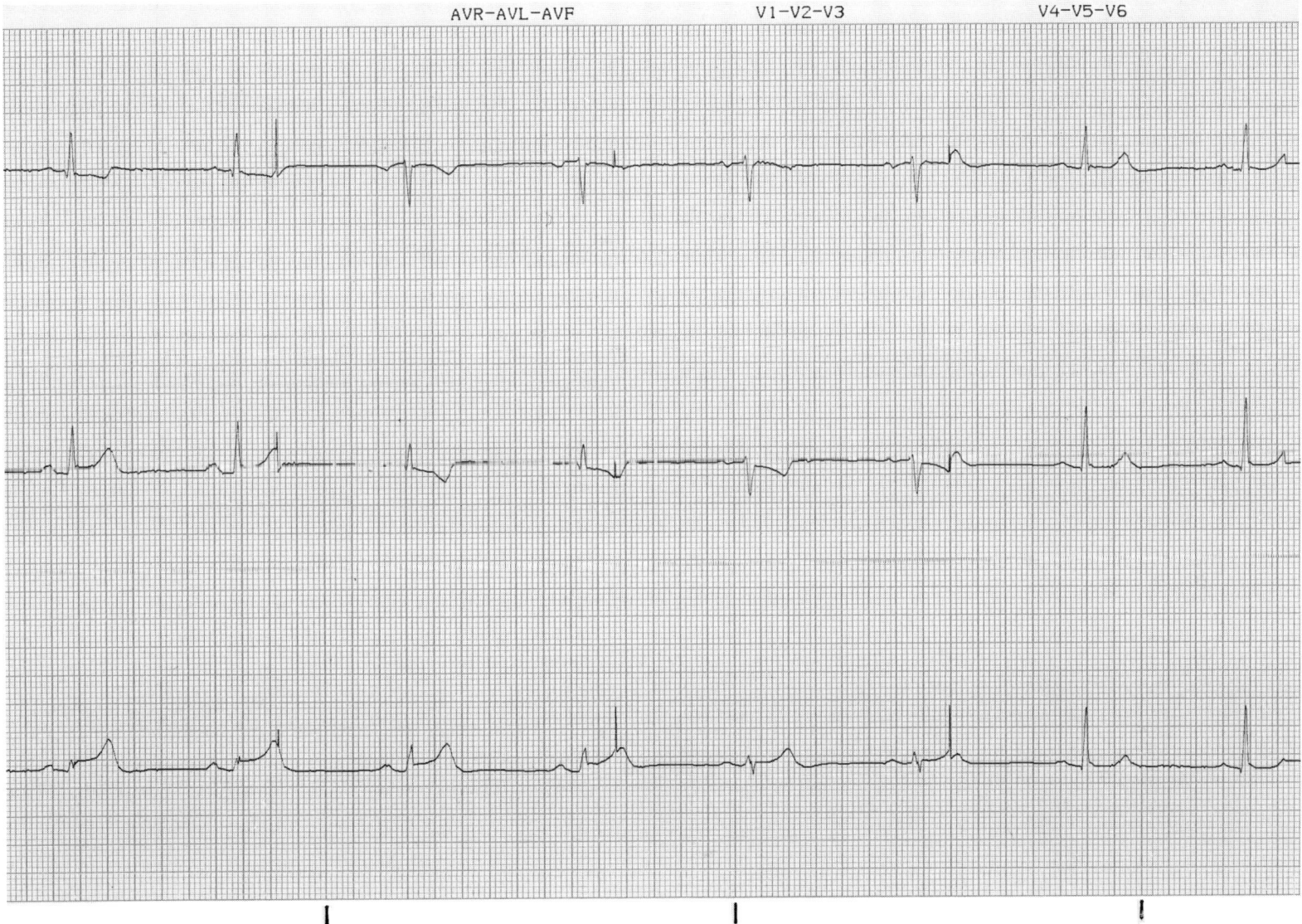

CASE 44

Rate and Rhythm

There is a P wave preceding each QRS complex, and the rhythm is normal sinus rhythm.

The heart rate is about 85 beats per minute.

Intervals

PR interval: 0.16s
QRS duration: 0.08s
QT interval: 0.36s

QRS Axis

The QRS complex is positive in lead I and negative in lead aVF, so the QRS axis is in the leftward quadrant. The isoelectric lead is II, so the QRS axis is −30 degrees. This is left axis deviation.

Evidence for Atrial Enlargement

There is no evidence for atrial enlargement.

Evidence for Ventricular Hypertrophy

LVH: The sum of the S wave in V1 (14 mm) and the R wave in V5 (8 mm) is 22 mm. There is no evidence of left ventricular hypertrophy by voltage criteria.

RVH: There is no evidence for right ventricular hypertrophy.

R-Wave Progression

The R waves grow slowly, and the QRS complex does not become mostly positive until V6. Thus there is poor R-wave progression.

Evidence of Ischemia or Infarction

Anterior leads: There is poor R-wave progression. There are also nonspecific ST-T wave abnormalities.

Inferior leads: There are no specific changes consistent with ischemia.

Summary

Normal sinus rhythm at 85 bpm
Intervals: 0.16/0.08/0.36
QRS axis: −30 degrees
Left axis deviation consistent with left anterior hemiblock
Poor R-wave progression consistent with anterior MI, clockwise rotation, or faulty lead placement

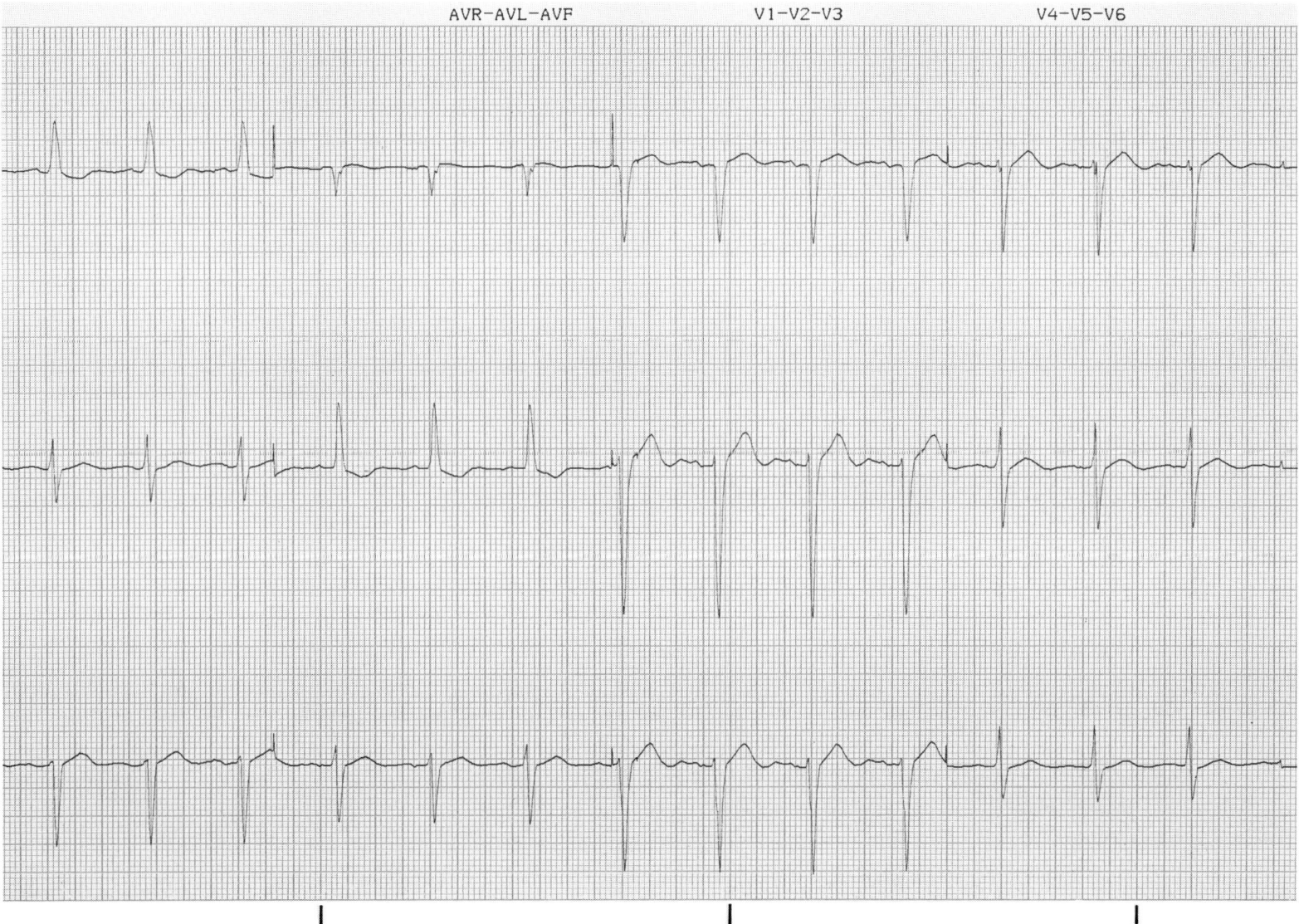

CASE 45

Rate and Rhythm

There is a P wave preceding each QRS complex, and the rhythm is normal sinus rhythm.

The heart rate is about 75 beats per minute.

Intervals

PR interval: 0.20s
QRS duration: 0.08s
QT interval: 0.40s

QRS Axis

The QRS complex is positive in lead I and positive in lead aVF, so the QRS axis is in the normal quadrant. Leads I and aVL are closest to isoelectric, so the QRS axis is between +60 and +90 degrees, or +75 degrees.

Evidence for Atrial Enlargement

In lead II, the P waves are notched and widened to more than 2.5 mm. In lead V1, the P waves are biphasic, with the terminal part wider than 1 mm. Thus there is left atrial enlargement.

Evidence for Ventricular Hypertrophy

LVH: The sum of the S wave in V1 (17 mm) and the R wave in V5 (15 mm) is 32 mm. This does not meet voltage criteria for left ventricular hypertrophy.

RVH: The QRS axis is in the normal quadrant. There is no evidence for right ventricular hypertrophy.

R-Wave Progression

The R waves grow slowly, and the QRS complex does not become mostly positive until V5. There is poor R-wave progression.

Evidence of Ischemia or Infarction

Anterior leads: There is downsloping ST-segment depression in V5 and V6 consistent with digoxin effect or apical ischemia or subendocardial infarction.

Inferior leads: There are no specific changes consistent with ischemia.

Summary

Normal sinus rhythm at 75 bpm
Intervals: 0.20/0.08/0.40
QRS axis: +75 degrees
Left atrial enlargement
Poor R-wave progression consistent with anterior MI, clockwise rotation, or faulty lead placement
ST-segment depression in V5 and V6 consistent with digoxin effect, but also with apical ischemia or subendocardial infarction

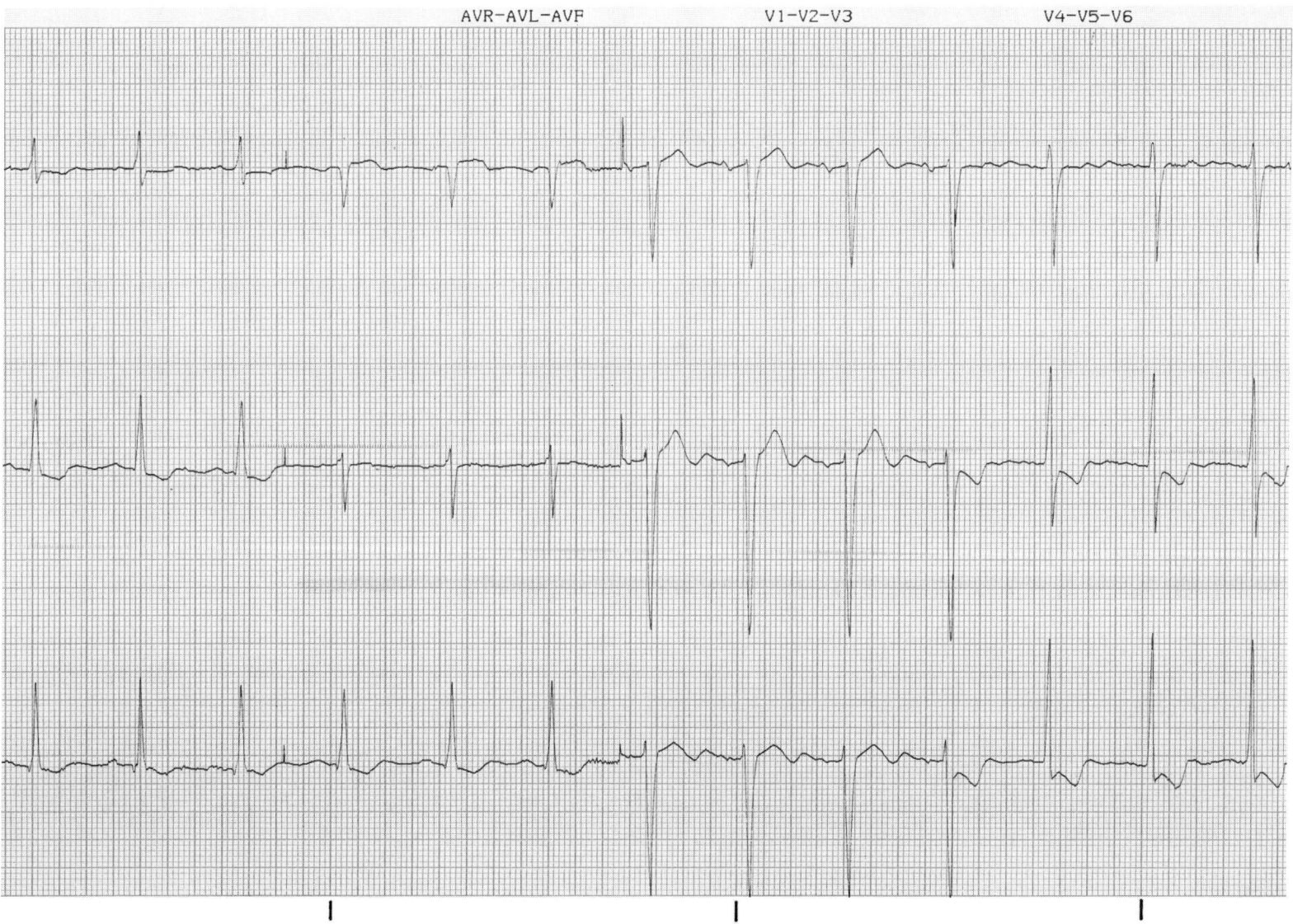

CASE 46

Rate and Rhythm

There is a P wave preceding each QRS complex, and the rhythm is normal sinus rhythm.

The heart rate is about 65 beats per minute.

Intervals

PR interval: 0.18s
QRS duration: 0.08s
QT interval: 0.40s

QRS Axis

The QRS complex is positive in lead I and isoelectric in lead aVF, so the QRS axis is about zero.

Evidence for Atrial Enlargement

There is no evidence for atrial enlargement.

Evidence for Ventricular Hypertrophy

LVH: The sum of the S wave in V1 (5 mm) and the R wave in V5 (4 mm) is 9 mm. There is no evidence of left ventricular hypertrophy by voltage criteria. In fact, there is low voltage, since the QRS complexes in the limb leads are 5 mm or less in width and the QRS complexes in the precordial leads are 15 mm or less in width.

RVH: The QRS axis is in the normal quadrant. There is no evidence for right ventricular hypertrophy.

R-Wave Progression

The R waves grow from V2 to V5, and the QRS complexes become mostly positive by V4, so the R-wave progression is close to normal.

Evidence of Ischemia or Infarction

Anterior leads: There are biphasic T waves in leads V3 to V6 and ST-segment depressions in aVL consistent with anterolateral ischemia or subendocardial infarction. The ST segments in V6 are elevated.

Inferior leads: There are ST-segment elevations in II, III, and aVF with Q waves in III and aVF consistent with acute inferior MI.

Summary

Normal sinus rhythm at 65 bpm
Intervals: 0.18/0.08/0.40
QRS axis: 0 degrees
Low voltage, raising the possibility of pericardial effusion, hypothyroidism, or chest wall abnormality
ST-segment elevation in II, III, aVF, and V6 with Q waves in III and aVF consistent with acute inferoapical MI
Biphasic T waves in V3 to V6 and ST-segment depression in aVL consistent with anterolateral ischemia or subendocardial infarction

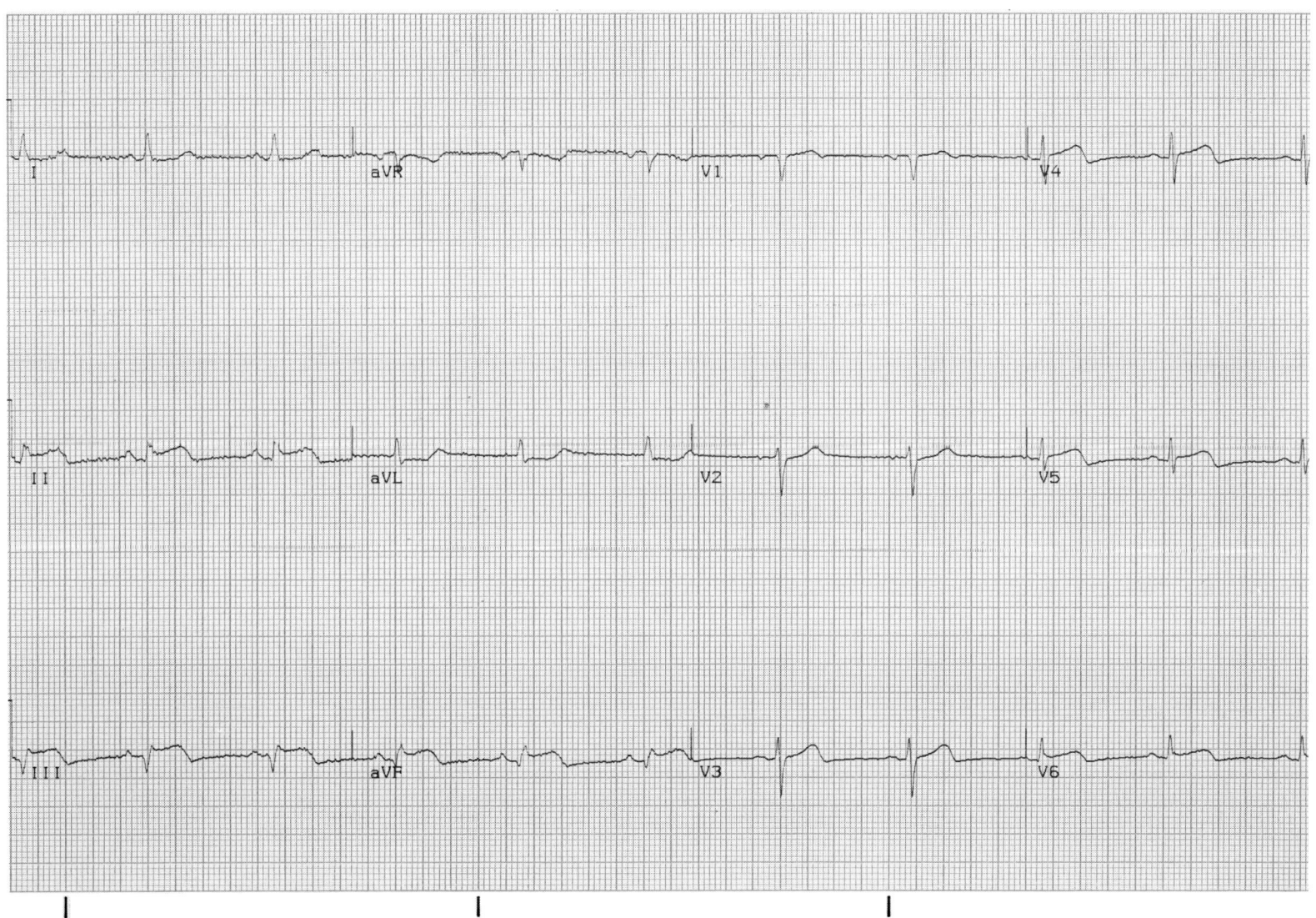

CASE 47

Rate and Rhythm

There is a P wave preceding each QRS complex, and the rhythm is normal sinus rhythm.

The heart rate is 80 beats per minute.

Intervals

PR interval: 0.20s
QRS duration: 0.10s
QT interval: 0.36s

The wide QRS duration indicates that there is an interventricular conduction delay. This accounts for the splintered appearance of the QRS complex in V3, II, and aVF.

QRS Axis

The QRS complex is positive in lead I and isoelectric in lead aVF, so the QRS axis is about zero.

Evidence for Atrial Enlargement

In lead II, the P waves are notched and widened to more than 2.5 mm. In lead V1, the P waves are biphasic, with the terminal part wider than 1 mm. Thus there is left atrial enlargement.

Evidence for Ventricular Hypertrophy

LVH: The sum of the S wave in V1 (19 mm) and the R wave in V5 (25 mm) is 44 mm. Thus there is left ventricular hypertrophy by voltage criteria. Note also that the QRS voltage in lead aVL is 11 mm or greater.
RVH: The QRS axis is about zero, and there is no evidence for right ventricular hypertrophy.

R-Wave Progression

The R waves grow from V1 to V5 and the QRS complex becomes mostly positive in V4, so there is normal R-wave progression.

Evidence of Ischemia or Infarction

Anterior leads: There are downsloping ST-segment depressions in leads V4 to V6, I, and aVL consistent with possible anterolateral ischemia. However, these changes are also consistent with left ventricular hypertrophy and digoxin effect.
Inferior leads: There are no specific changes suggestive of ischemia.

Summary

Normal sinus rhythm at 80 bpm
Intervals: 0.20/0.10/0.36
QRS axis: 0 degrees
Interventricular conduction delay
Left atrial enlargement
Left ventricular hypertrophy
ST-segment depression in V4 to V6, I, and aVL consistent with left ventricular hypertrophy, digoxin effect, or anterior ischemia

CASE 47

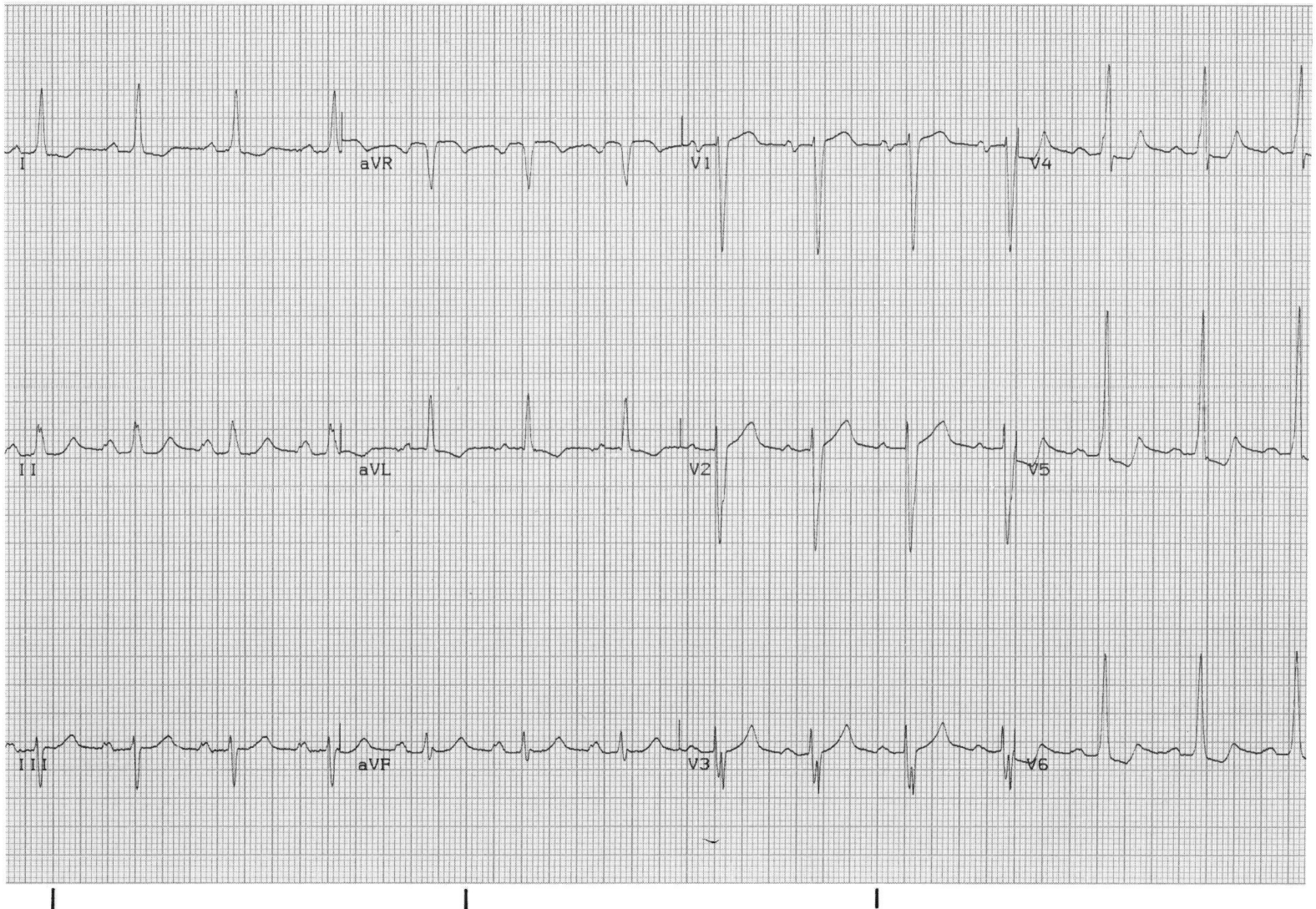

CASE 48

Rate and Rhythm

There is a P wave preceding each QRS complex, and the rhythm is normal sinus rhythm.

The heart rate is about 65 beats per minute.

Intervals

PR interval: 0.32s
QRS duration: 0.08s
QT interval: 0.40s

The PR interval is very prolonged, indicating that there is a marked first-degree AV block. Notice that the QRS complex in lead V1 has an RSR' morphology, even though the QRS duration is not prolonged. This is an incomplete right bundle-branch block pattern in V1, which is a normal variant. It is sometimes called a *crista terminalis pattern*.

QRS Axis

The QRS complex is positive in lead I and negative in lead aVF, so the QRS axis is in the leftward quadrant. The isoelectric lead is II, so the QRS axis is −30 degrees. This is left axis deviation.

Evidence for Atrial Enlargement

In lead II, the P waves are notched, but they are not widened to 2.5 mm. There is no evidence for atrial enlargement.

Evidence for Ventricular Hypertrophy

LVH: The sum of the S wave in V1 (16 mm) and the R wave in V5 (21 mm) is 37 mm. Thus there is left ventricular hypertrophy by voltage criteria. Notice that the QRS voltage is greater than 11 mm in lead aVL. In the setting of left ventricular hypertrophy, left axis deviation may be secondary to the ventricular hypertrophy.

RVH: The QRS axis is in the leftward quadrant. There is no evidence for right ventricular hypertrophy.

R-Wave Progression

The R waves do not grow from V1 to V2, and the QRS complexes do not become mostly positive until V5. There is poor R-wave progression.

Evidence of Ischemia or Infarction

Anterior leads: There is poor R-wave progression and ST-segment depression and T-wave inversion in V5 and V6.

Inferior leads: There are ST-segment depressions and T-wave inversions in II, III, and aVF.

ST-T waves: We know that there is left ventricular hypertrophy. The changes in the apical and inferior leads are consistent with secondary changes from left ventricular hypertrophy, as is the left axis deviation. Thus we need not postulate other causes for these changes (that is, inferoapical ischemia to explain the ST-T wave changes or left anterior hemiblock to explain the left axis deviation).

Summary

Normal sinus rhythm at 65 bpm, with marked first-degree AV block
Intervals: 0.32/0.08/0.40
QRS axis: −30 degrees
Incomplete right bundle-branch block pattern in V1, normal variant
Poor R-wave progression
Left ventricular hypertrophy with left axis deviation and secondary ST-T wave changes

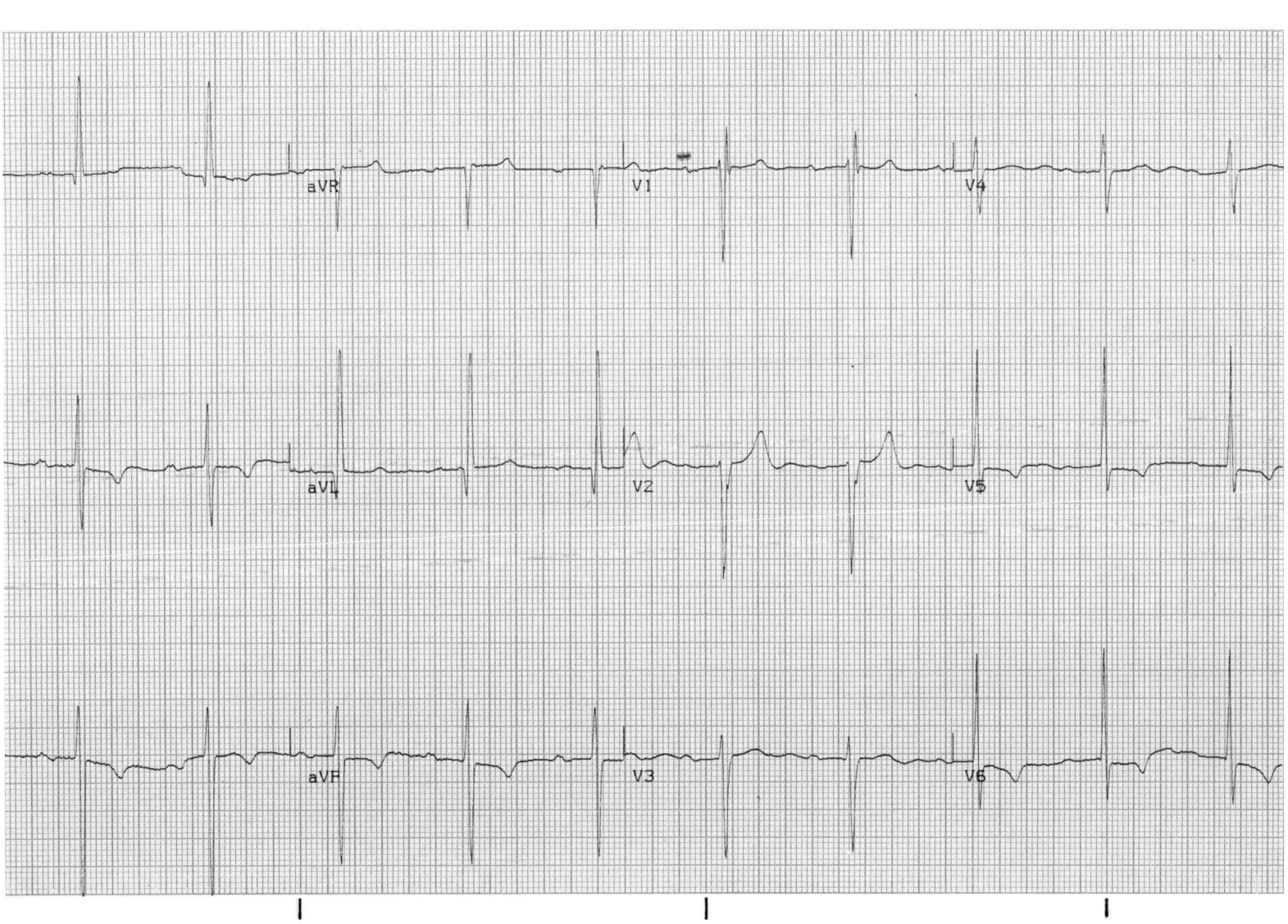

CASE 49

Rate and Rhythm

There is a P wave preceding each QRS complex, and the rhythm is normal sinus rhythm.

The heart rate is 70 beats per minute.

Intervals

PR interval: 0.20s
QRS duration: 0.08s
QT interval: 0.32s

QRS Axis

The QRS complex is positive in lead I and isoelectric in lead aVF, so the QRS axis is about zero.

Evidence for Atrial Enlargement

There is no evidence for atrial enlargement.

Evidence for Ventricular Hypertrophy

LVH: The sum of the S wave in V1 (12 mm) and the R wave in V6 (10 mm) is 22 mm. There is no evidence of left ventricular hypertrophy by voltage criteria.
RVH: The QRS axis is zero, and there is no evidence for right ventricular hypertrophy.

R-Wave Progression

There are Q waves in V1 to V5, so there is poor R-wave progression.

Evidence of Ischemia or Infarction

Anterior leads: There are Q waves and ST-segment elevations in V1 to V5 consistent with acute anterior MI. There are T-wave inversions in I and aVL consistent with lateral ischemia or subendocardial infarction.
Inferior leads: There are significant Q waves in II and aVF consistent with inferior MI. Unlike in the anterior leads, there are no ST-segment elevations, so the age of the inferior MI is unknown.

Summary

Normal sinus rhythm at 70 bpm
Intervals: 0.20/0.08/0.32
QRS axis: 0 degrees
ST-segment elevations and Q waves in V1 to V5 consistent with acute anterior MI
ST-segment depression in I and aVL consistent with lateral ischemia or subendocardial infarction
Q waves in II and aVF consistent with inferior MI of indeterminate age

CASE 49

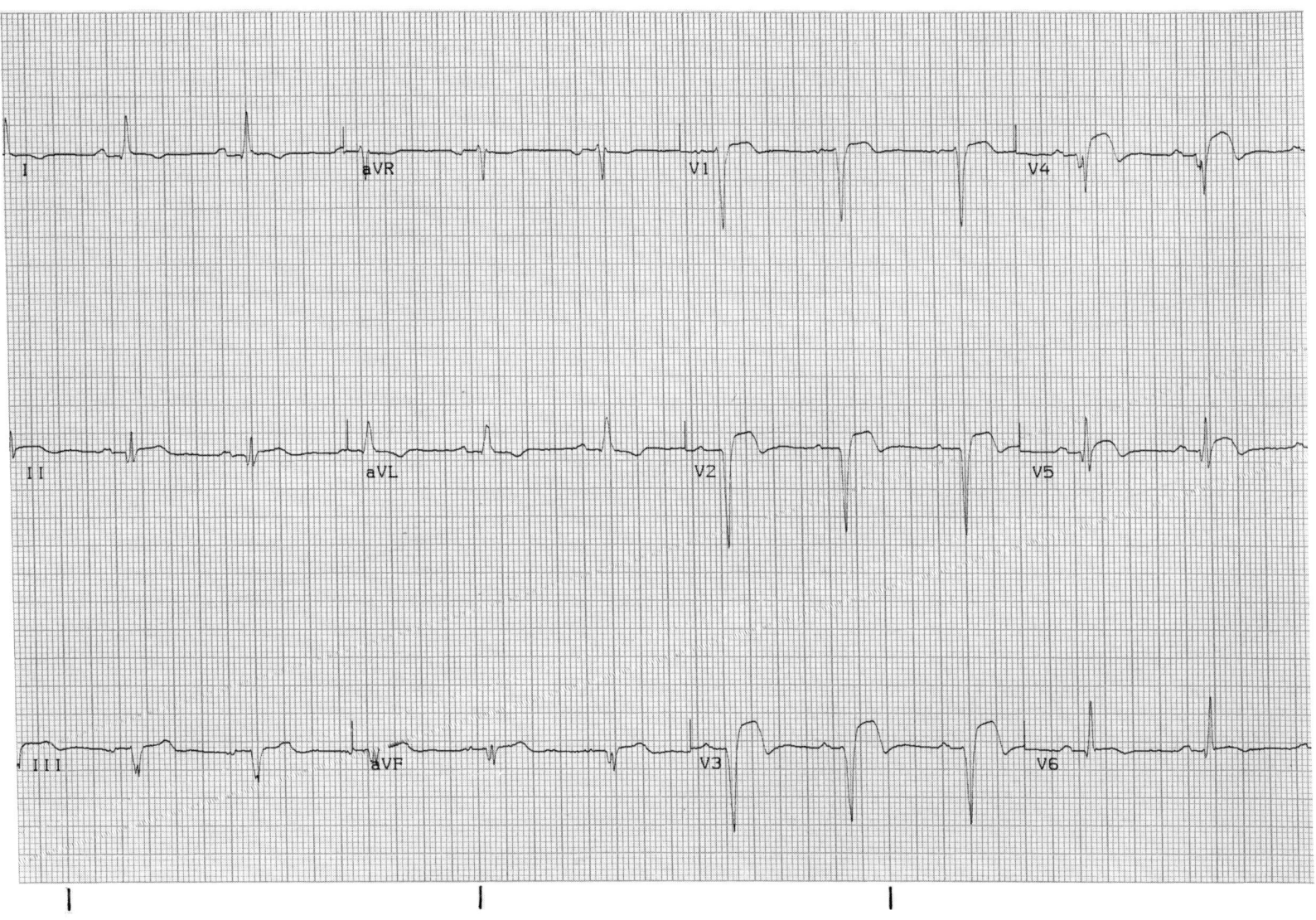

CASE 50

Rate and Rhythm

There is a P wave preceding each QRS complex, and the rhythm is sinus tachycardia.

The heart rate is about 105 beats per minute.

Intervals

PR interval: 0.20s
QRS duration: 0.12s
QT interval: 0.32s

The prolonged QRS duration indicates a bundle-branch block. Examination of the QRS complex in lead V1 shows the RSR' pattern typical of right bundle-branch block.

QRS Axis

The QRS complex is negative in lead I and isoelectric in lead aVF, so the QRS axis is about +180 degrees. This is extreme right axis deviation.

Evidence for Atrial Enlargement

In lead II, the P waves are tall, measuring greater than 2.5 mm in height as well as in width. In V1, the P waves are difficult to distinguish from the T waves, but they are biphasic, with the first part greater than 1 mm. Thus there is certainly right atrial enlargement and possibly left atrial enlargement as well.

Evidence for Ventricular Hypertrophy

LVH: The sum of the S wave in V1 (4 mm) and the R wave in V5 (14 mm) is 18 mm. This does not meet voltage criteria for left ventricular hypertrophy.

RVH: The QRS axis is +180 degrees, showing extreme right axis deviation. With right bundle-branch block, it is difficult to assess voltage criteria for right ventricular hypertrophy, since the R' that represents the right ventricle is broad and its voltage unreliable. Still, the pattern in V6 is not typical for right bundle-branch block, and the R/S ratio there is less than 1. There is probably right ventricular hypertrophy.

R-Wave Progression

There is a Q wave in V2, and there is little R-wave growth from V1 to V3. Thus there is poor R-wave progression.

Evidence of Ischemia or Infarction

Anterior leads: There is poor R-wave progression with a Q wave in V2. There are no other changes to indicate anterior ischemia or infarction.

Inferior leads: There are no specific changes of ischemia or infarction.

ST-T waves: There are ST-T wave changes secondary to right bundle-branch block and possibly right ventricular hypertrophy.

Summary

Sinus tachycardia at 105 bpm
Intervals: 0.20/0.12/0.32
QRS axis: +180 degrees
Right axis deviation
Right bundle-branch block
Right atrial enlargement and possible left atrial enlargement
Probable right ventricular hypertrophy

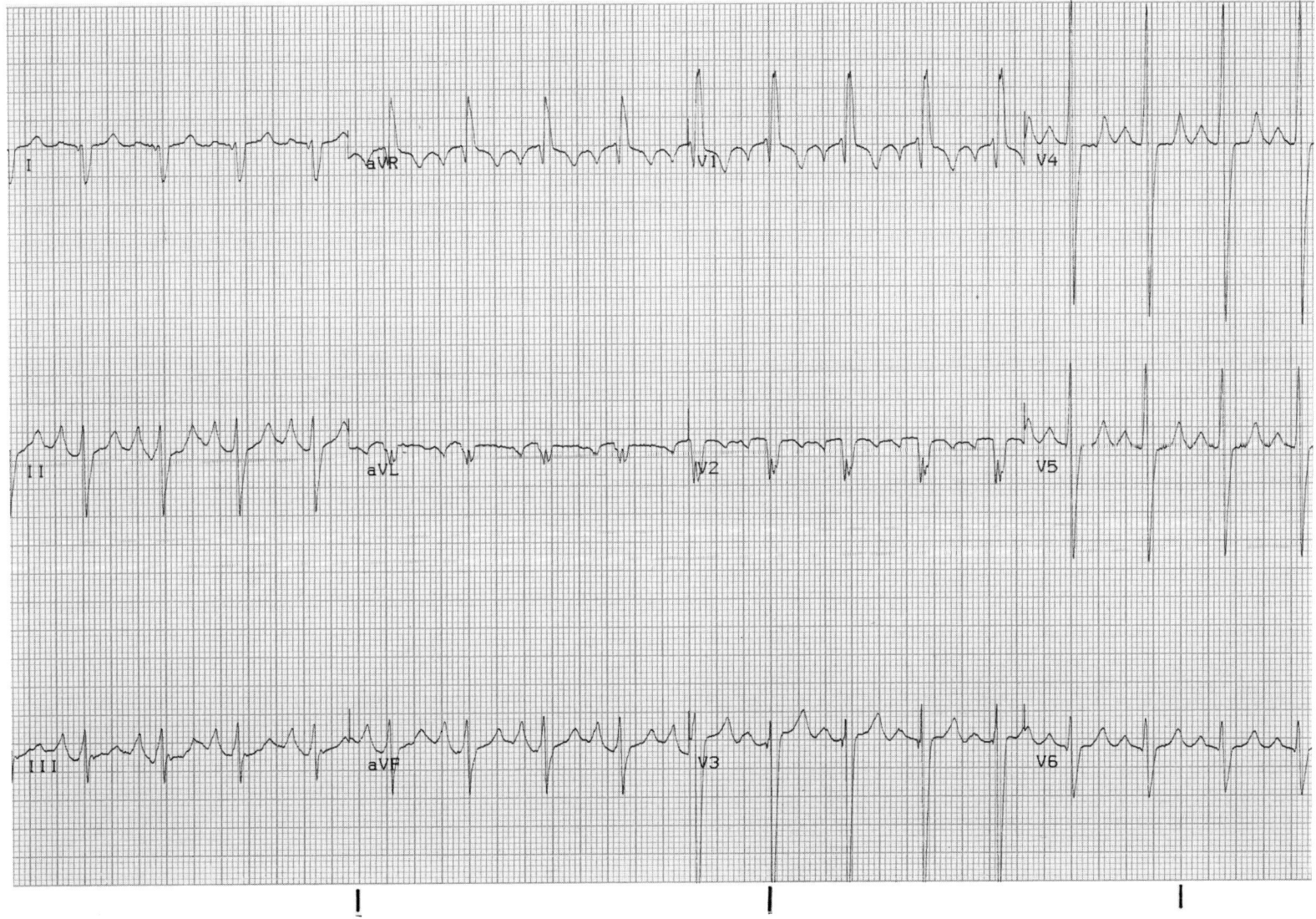

CASE 51

Rate and Rhythm

There is a P wave preceding each QRS complex, and the rhythm is normal sinus rhythm.

The heart rate is about 75 beats per minute.

Intervals

PR interval: 0.12s
QRS duration: 0.08s
QT interval: 0.36s

QRS Axis

The QRS complex is positive in lead I and positive in lead aVF, so the QRS axis is in the normal quadrant. The isoelectric lead is III, so the QRS axis is about +30 degrees.

Evidence for Atrial Enlargement

There is no evidence for atrial enlargement.

Evidence for Ventricular Hypertrophy

LVH: The sum of the S wave in V1 (25 mm) and the R wave in V5 (15 mm) is 40 mm. While this meets voltage criteria for left ventricular hypertrophy, these voltages would be normal in a person less than 35 years old.

RVH: The QRS axis is in the normal quadrant. There is no evidence for right ventricular hypertrophy.

R-Wave Progression

The R waves grow from V1 to V4, and the QRS complex becomes mostly positive in V3. Thus there is good (normal) R-wave progression.

Evidence of Ischemia or Infarction

Anterior leads: There is no specific evidence of anterior ischemia.
Inferior leads: There is no specific evidence of inferior ischemia.
ST-T waves: There is normal early repolarization seen best in V5, V6, II, and aVF. These changes are a normal variant and are not a cause for concern in a young person.

Summary

Normal sinus rhythm at 75 bpm
Intervals: 0.12/0.08/0.36
QRS axis: +30 degrees
Normal early repolarization
Tracing within normal limits

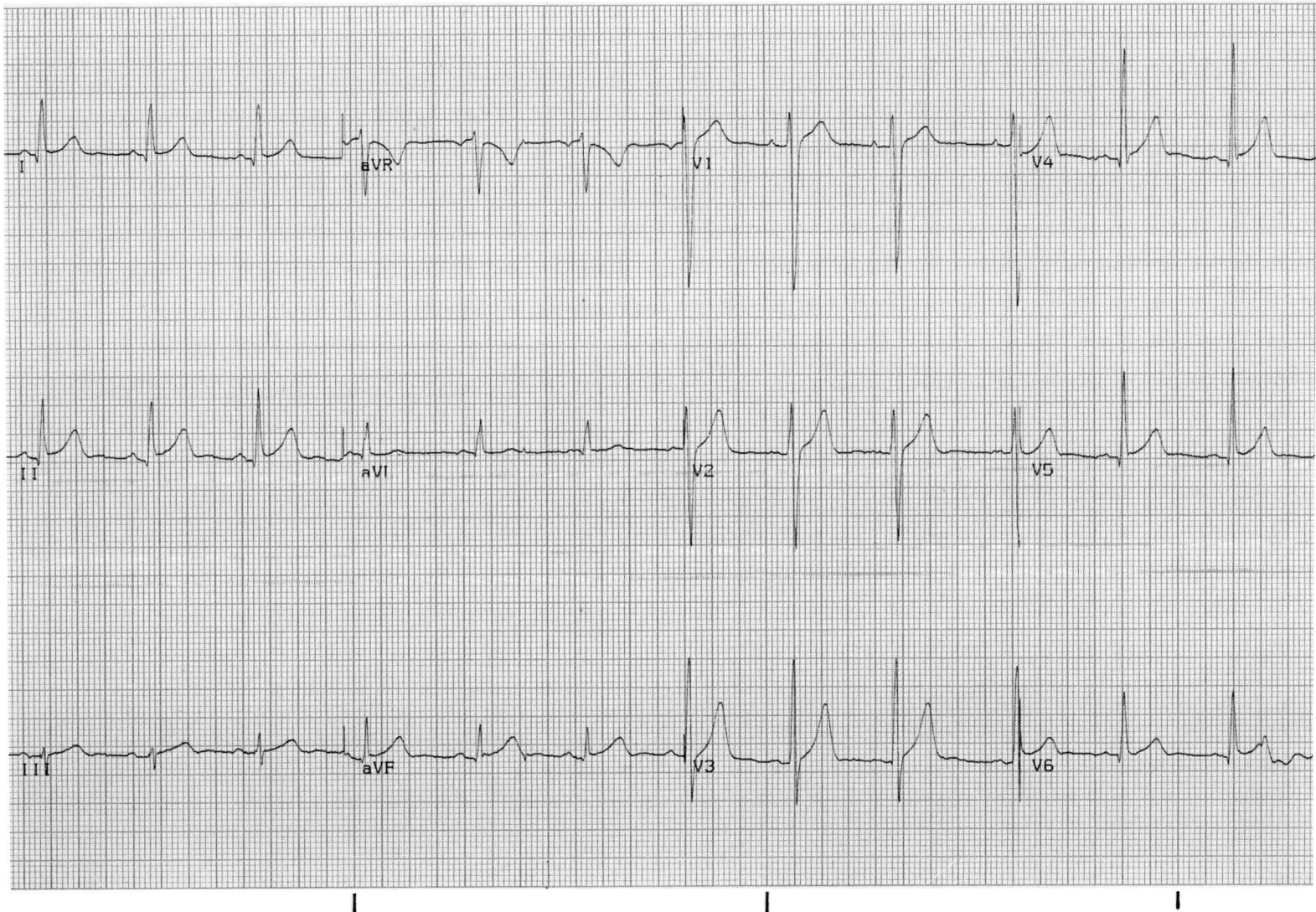

CASE 52

Rate and Rhythm

The rhythm is irregular, and there are no P waves. This is atrial fibrillation. Using the 6-s method to estimate rates, the ventricular rate is about 100 beats per minute. Thus this is atrial fibrillation with moderate to rapid ventricular response. There is one wide complex QRS complex, which probably represents a premature ventricular contraction.

Intervals

PR interval: not applicable
QRS duration: 0.06s
QT interval: 0.36s

QRS Axis

The QRS complex is positive in lead I and negative in lead aVF, so the QRS axis is in the leftward quadrant. The isoelectric lead is II, so the QRS axis is −30 degrees. This is left axis deviation.

Evidence for Atrial Enlargement

There are no P waves, so we cannot assess for atrial enlargement.

Evidence for Ventricular Hypertrophy

LVH: The sum of the S wave in V1 (10 mm) and the R wave in V5 (21) is 31 mm. This does not meet voltage criteria for left ventricular hypertrophy.

RVH: The QRS axis is in the leftward quadrant. There is no evidence for right ventricular hypertrophy.

R-Wave Progression

The R waves grow very little from V1 to V4. There is poor R-wave progression, consistent with clockwise rotation, faulty lead placement, or anterior MI.

Evidence of Ischemia or Infarction

Anterior leads: There is poor R-wave progression. There is ST-segment depression in V5 and V6 consistent with apical ischemia or digoxin effect.
Inferior leads: There are no specific changes of inferior ischemia or infarction.
ST-T waves: There are nonspecific ST-T wave abnormalities.

Summary

Atrial fibrillation with moderate to rapid ventricular response, with one premature ventricular beat
Intervals: n.a./0.06/0.36
QRS axis: −30 degrees
Left axis deviation consistent with left anterior hemiblock
Poor R-wave progression consistent with anterior MI, clockwise rotation, or faulty lead placement
ST-segment depression in V5 and V6 consistent with digoxin effect or apical ischemia
Nonspecific ST-T wave abnormalities

CASE 52

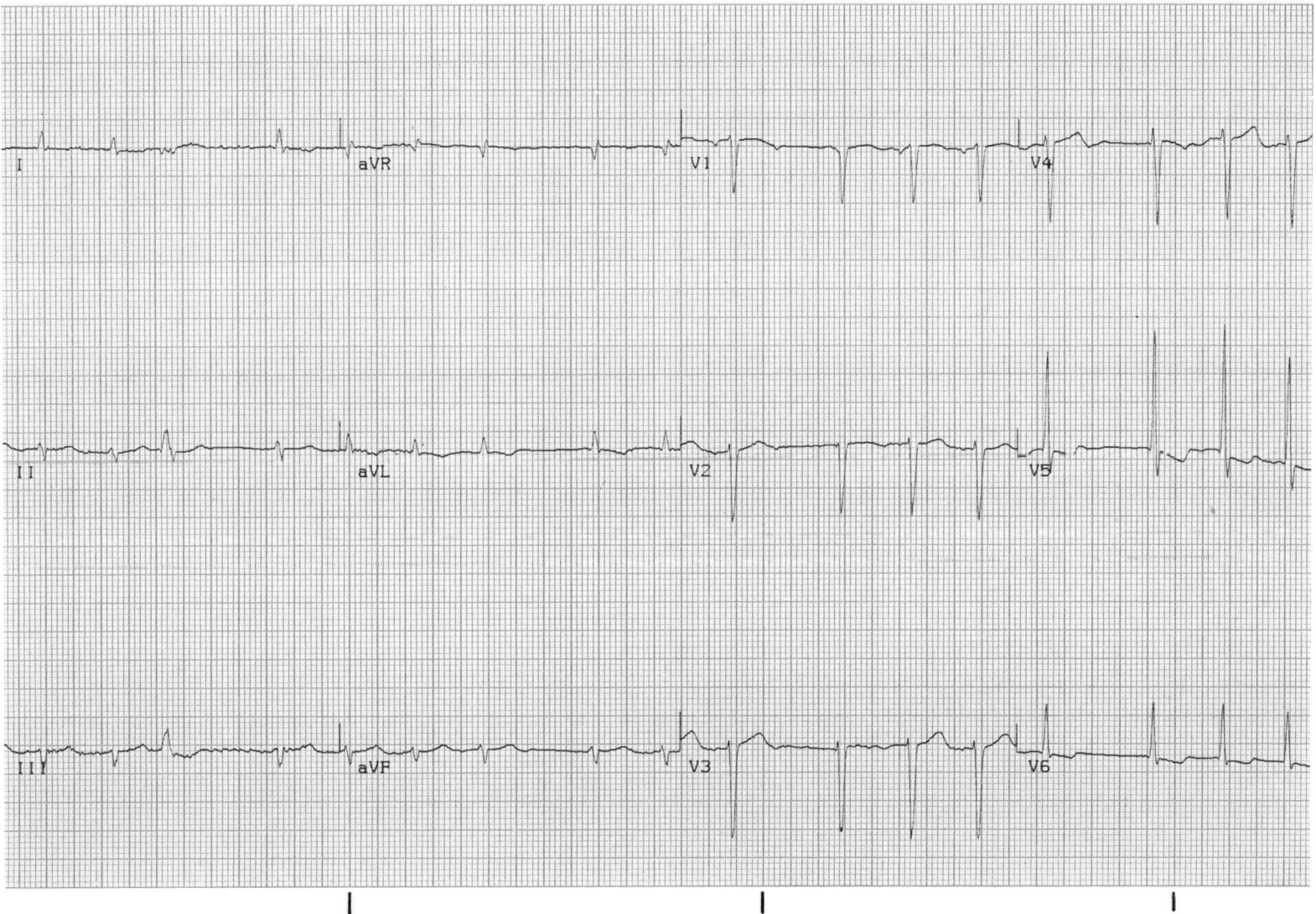

CASE 53

Rate and Rhythm

There is a P wave preceding each QRS complex, and the rhythm is normal sinus rhythm.

The heart rate is about 90 beats per minute.

Intervals

PR interval: 0.18s
QRS duration: 0.08s
QT interval: 0.36s

The QRS duration is normal, but the QRS complex in V1 shows an incomplete right bundle-branch block. This is a normal variant.

QRS Axis

The QRS complex is positive in lead I and positive in lead aVF, so the QRS axis is in the normal quadrant. Leads aVL and III are closest to isoelectric, so the QRS axis is between +60 and +30 degrees, or about +45 degrees.

Evidence for Atrial Enlargement

In lead II, the P waves are notched and widened to more than 2.5 mm. In lead V1, the P waves are biphasic, with the terminal part wider than 1 mm. Thus there is left atrial enlargement.

Evidence for Ventricular Hypertrophy

LVH: The sum of the S wave in V1 (7 mm) and the R wave in V5 (14 mm) is 21 mm. There is no evidence of left ventricular hypertrophy by voltage criteria.
RVH: The QRS axis is in the normal quadrant. There is no evidence for right ventricular hypertrophy.

R-Wave Progression

The R waves grow normally from V1 to V5, and the QRS complex becomes mostly positive in V3. Thus there is normal R-wave progression.

Evidence of Ischemia or Infarction

Anterior leads: There are no changes consistent with anterior ischemia or infarction.
Inferior leads: There are no changes consistent with inferior ischemia or infarction.

Summary

Normal sinus rhythm at 90 bpm
Intervals: 0.18/0.08/0.36
QRS axis: +45 degrees
Left atrial enlargement

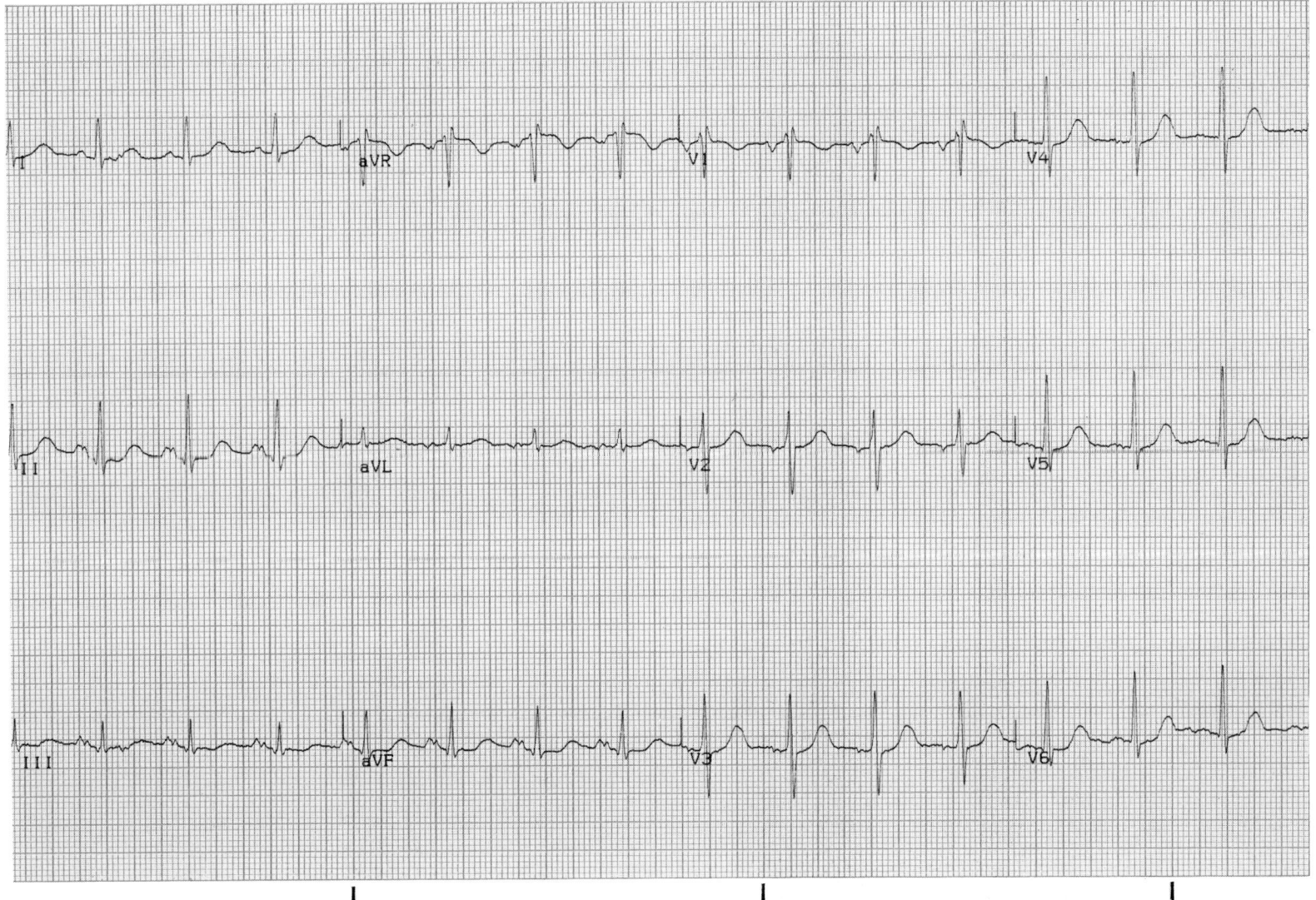

CASE 54

Rate and Rhythm

There is a P wave preceding each QRS complex, and the rhythm is normal sinus rhythm.

The heart rate is about 80 beats per minute.

Intervals

PR interval: 0.18s
QRS duration: 0.06s
QT interval: 0.36s

QRS Axis

The QRS complex is positive in lead I and positive in lead aVF, so the QRS axis is in the normal quadrant. The isoelectric lead is III, so the QRS axis is +30 degrees.

Evidence for Atrial Enlargement

In lead II, the P waves are widened to more than 2.5 mm. In lead V1, the P waves are biphasic, with the terminal part measuring 1 mm. These changes are suggestive of left atrial enlargement.

Evidence for Ventricular Hypertrophy

LVH: The sum of the S wave in V1 (10 mm) and the R wave in V5 (14 m) is 24 mm. There is no evidence of left ventricular hypertrophy by voltage criteria.

RVH: The QRS axis is in the normal quadrant. There is no evidence for right ventricular hypertrophy.

R-Wave Progression

The R waves grow normally from V1 to V5, and the QRS complex becomes mostly positive in V3 and V4. Thus there is normal (good) R-wave progression.

Evidence of Ischemia or Infarction

Anterior leads: There are no changes that suggest anterior ischemia or infarction.

Inferior leads: There are no changes that suggest inferior ischemia or infarction. There is an isolated Q wave in III, which is a normal variant.

Summary

Normal sinus rhythm at 80 bpm
Intervals: 0.18/0.06/0.36
QRS axis: +30 degrees
Left atrial enlargement

CASE 54 □ 171

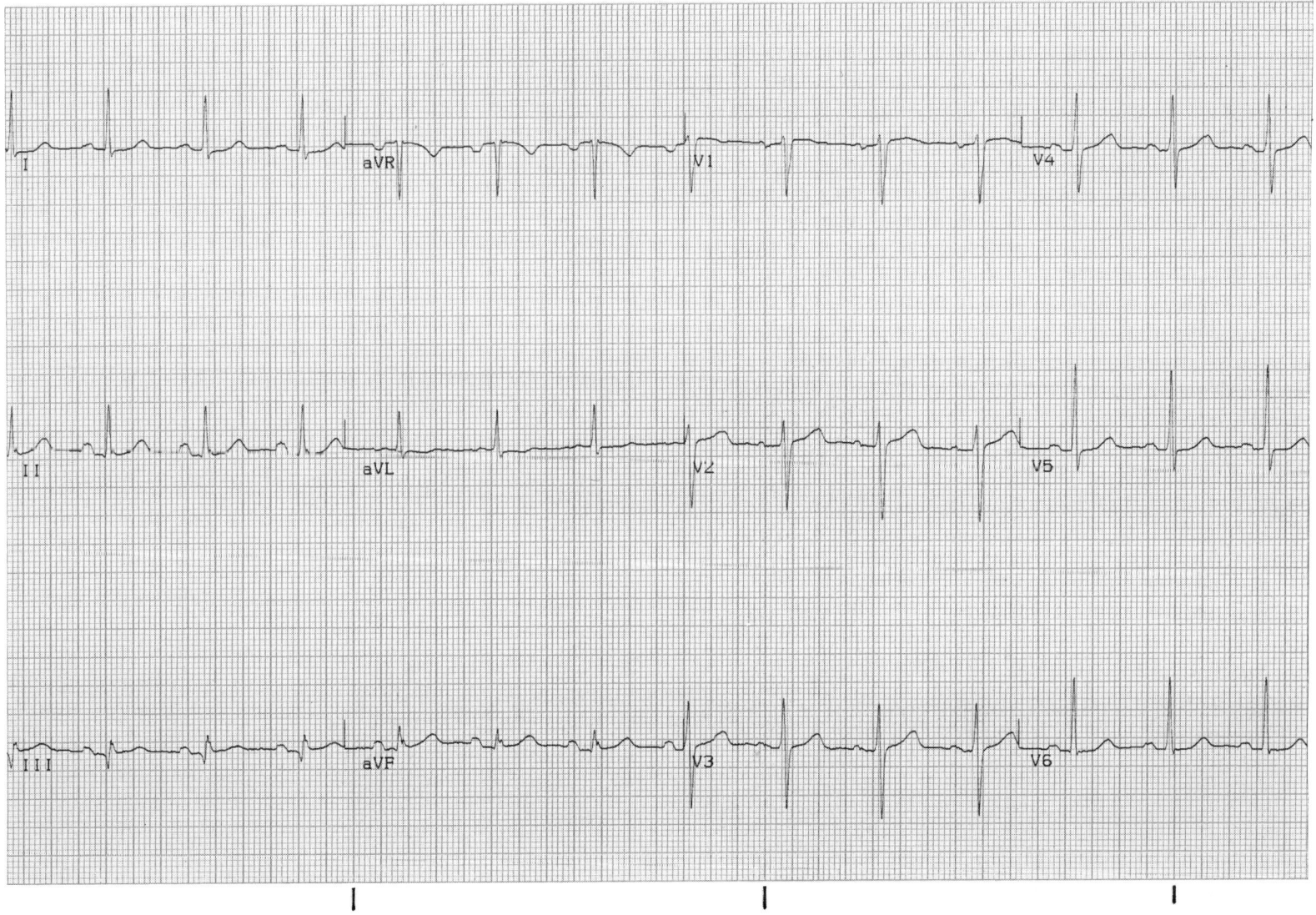

CASE 55

Rate and Rhythm

There is a P wave preceding each QRS complex, and the rhythm is sinus bradycardia.

The heart rate is between 50 and 55 beats per minute.

Intervals

PR interval: 0.16s
QRS duration: 0.12s
QT interval: 0.44s

The prolonged QRS duration indicates a bundle branch block. Examination of V1 shows the RSR' morphology typical of right bundle-branch block.

QRS Axis

The QRS complex is positive in lead I and positive in lead aVF, so the QRS axis is in the normal quadrant. The isoelectric lead is III, so the QRS axis is +30 degrees.

Evidence for Atrial Enlargement

There is no evidence for atrial enlargement.

Evidence for Ventricular Hypertrophy

LVH: The sum of the S wave in V1 (6 mm) and the R wave in V6 (12 mm) is 18 mm. There is no evidence of left ventricular hypertrophy by voltage criteria.
RVH: The QRS axis is in the normal quadrant. There is no evidence for right ventricular hypertrophy.

R-Wave Progression

The R waves grow from V1 to V6, and QRS complex becomes positive in V3. Thus the R-wave progression appears normal.

Evidence of Ischemia or Infarction

Anterior leads: There are no changes suggestive of anterior ischemia or infarction.
Inferior leads: There are no changes suggestive of inferior ischemia or infarction.
ST-T waves: There are ST-T wave changes that are secondary to the right bundle-branch block.

Summary

Sinus bradycardia at 55 bpm
Intervals: 0.16/0.12/0.44
QRS axis: +30 degrees
Right bundle-branch block

CASE 55 173

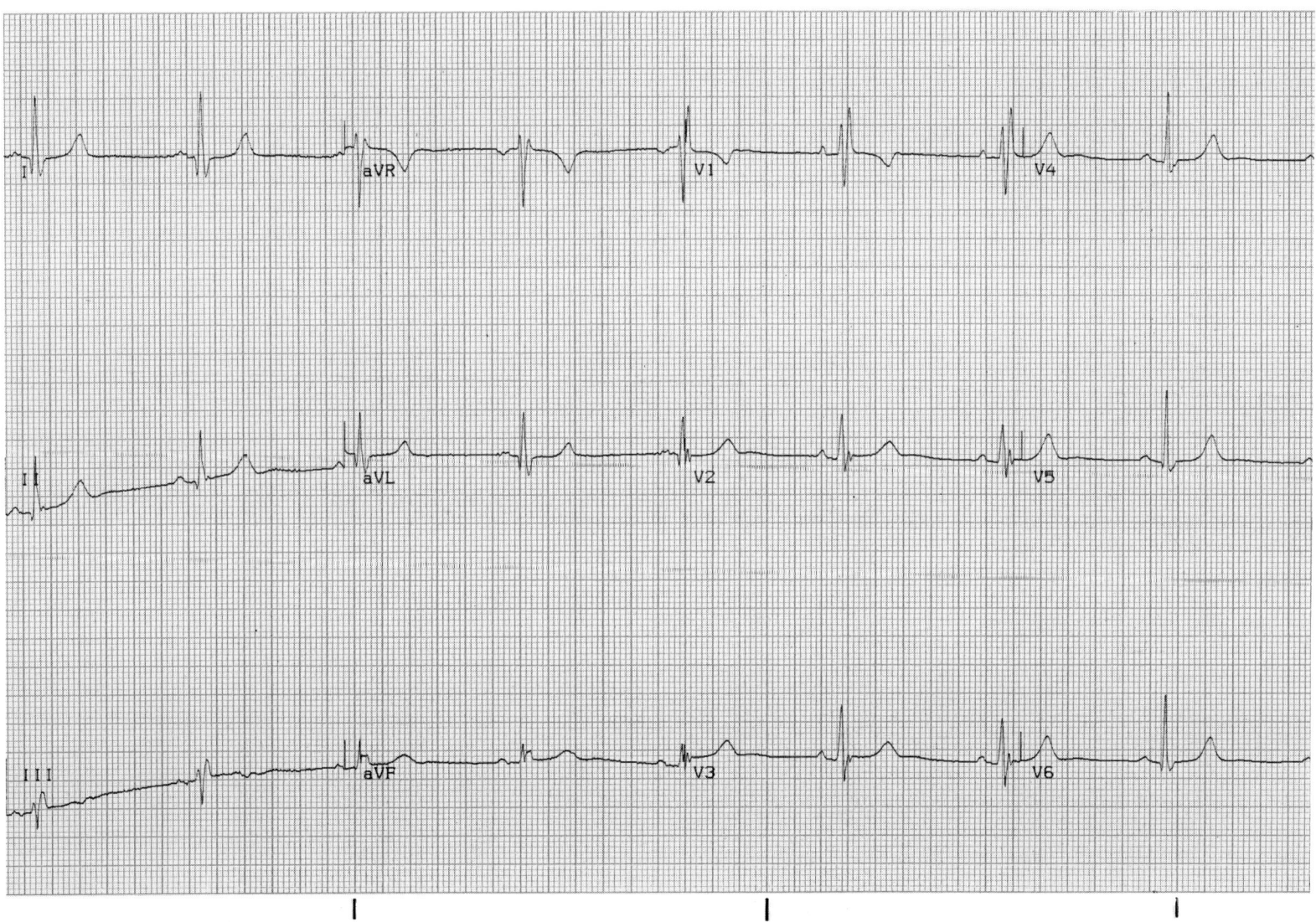

CASE 56

Rate and Rhythm

There is a P wave preceding each QRS complex, and the rhythm is sinus bradycardia. The heart rate is 50 beats per minute.

Intervals

PR interval: 0.16s
QRS duration: 0.06s
QT interval: 0.44s

QRS Axis

The QRS complex is positive in lead I, and positive in lead aV$_F$, so the QRS axis is in the normal quadrant. Leads III and aVL are closest to isoelectric, so the QRS axis is between +30 and +60 degrees, or about +45 degrees.

Evidence for Atrial Enlargement

There is no evidence for atrial enlargement.

Evidence for Ventricular Hypertrophy

LVH: The sum of the S wave in V1 (2 mm) and the R wave in V5 (21 mm) is 23 mm. There is no evidence of left ventricular hypertrophy by voltage criteria.

RVH: The QRS axis is in the normal quadrant. There is no evidence for right ventricular hypertrophy.

R-Wave Progression

The R waves grow in size from V1 to V6, and the QRS complex becomes mostly positive in V4. The R-wave progression is normal.

Evidence of Ischemia or Infarction

Anterior leads: There are inverted T waves in V4 to V6, consistent with anteroapical ischemia or subendocardial infarction.

Inferior leads: There are nonspecific ST-T wave abnormalities.

Summary

Sinus bradycardia at 50 bpm
Intervals: 0.16/0.06/0.44
QRS axis: +45 degrees
T-wave inversion in V4 to V6 consistent with anterior ischemia or subendocardial infarction
Nonspecific ST-T wave abnormalities

CASE 56

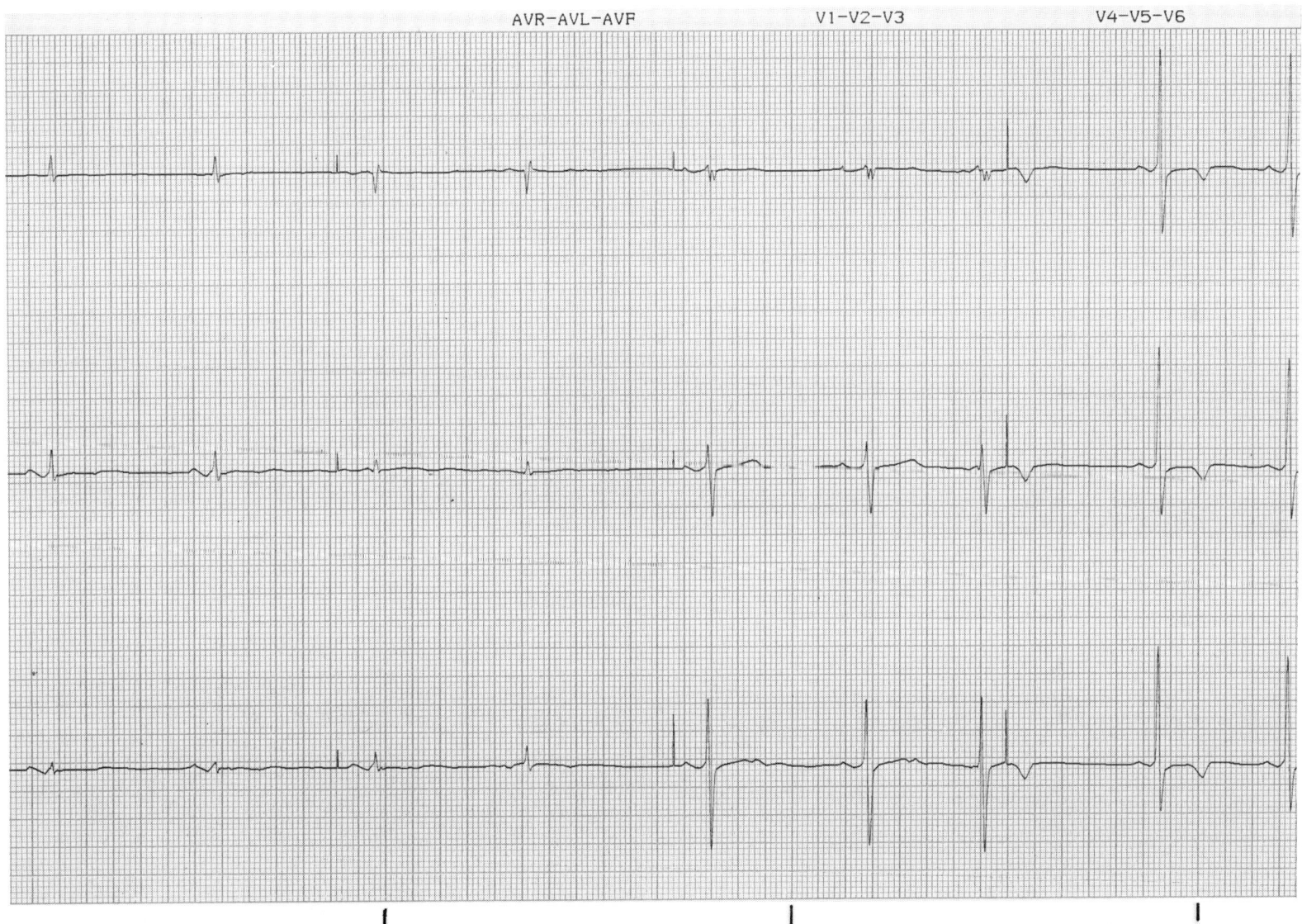

CASE 57

Rate and Rhythm

There are P waves preceding the QRS complexes, but the rhythm is irregular. Closer examination reveals that the P-wave morphologies are variable; in lead II, there are at least three different P-wave morphologies. The rhythm is multifocal atrial tachycardia.

Intervals

PR interval: not applicable
QRS duration: 0.06s
QT interval: 0.32s

QRS Axis

The QRS complex is positive in lead I and positive in lead aVF, so the QRS axis is in the normal quadrant. Leads III and aVF are closest to isoelectric, so the QRS axis is between 0 and +30 degrees, or about +15 degrees.

Evidence for Atrial Enlargement

Since we cannot tell which P wave originates from the sinus node, we cannot assess for atrial enlargement.

Evidence for Ventricular Hypertrophy

LVH: The sum of the S wave in V1 (12 mm) and the R wave in V6 (15 mm) is 27 mm. There is no evidence of left ventricular hypertrophy by voltage criteria.
RVH: The QRS axis is in the normal quadrant. There is no evidence for right ventricular hypertrophy.

R-Wave Progression

The R waves grow from V1 to V6, and the QRS complex becomes mostly positive in V4. There is normal R-wave progression.

Evidence of Ischemia or Infarction

Anterior leads: There are no definitive changes of ischemia or infarction.
Inferior leads: There are no definitive changes of ischemia or infarction.
ST-T waves: There are nonspecific ST-T wave abnormalities.

Summary

Multifocal atrial tachycardia
Intervals: n.a./0.06/0.32
QRS axis: +15 degrees
Nonspecific ST-T wave abnormalities

CASE 57 □ 177

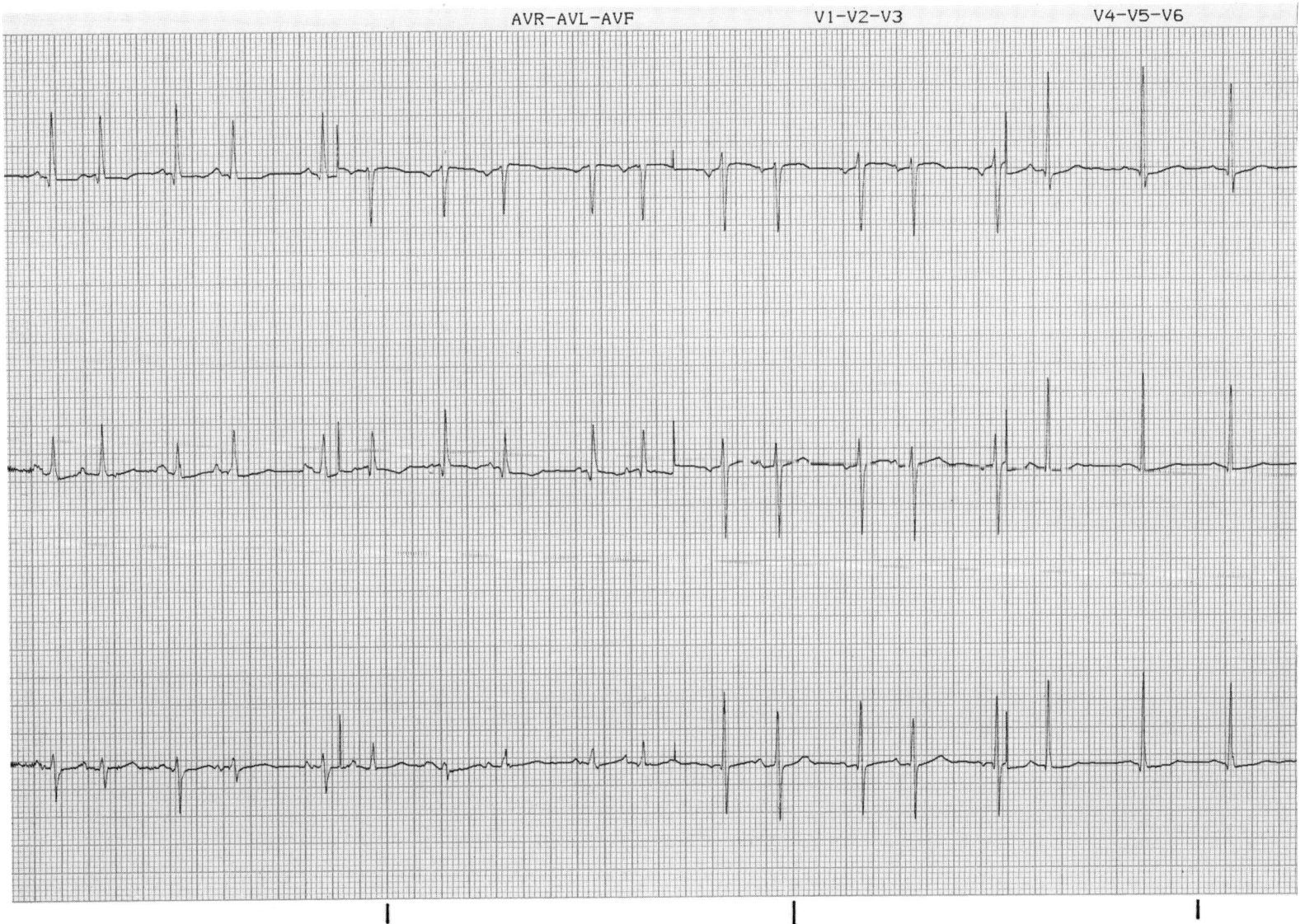

CASE 58

Rate and Rhythm

There is a P wave preceding each QRS complex, and the rhythm is normal sinus rhythm.

The heart rate is 90 beats per minute.

Intervals

PR interval: 0.16s
QRS duration: 0.08s
QT interval: 0.40s

QRS Axis

The QRS complex is positive in lead I and negative in lead aVF, so the QRS axis is in the leftward quadrant. The isoelectric lead is II, so the QRS axis is −30 degrees. This is left axis deviation, consistent with left anterior hemiblock.

Evidence for Atrial Enlargement

In lead II, the P waves are notched and widened to more than 2.5 mm. In lead V1, the P waves are biphasic, with the terminal part wider than 1 mm. Thus there is left atrial enlargement.

Evidence for Ventricular Hypertrophy

LVH: The sum of the S wave in V1 (9 mm) and the R wave in V6 (11 mm) is 20 mm. There is no evidence of left ventricular hypertrophy by voltage criteria.
RVH: The QRS axis is in the normal quadrant. There is no evidence for right ventricular hypertrophy.

R-Wave Progression

The R waves grow normally from V1 to V6, and the QRS complexes become mostly positive between V4 and V5. This is close to normal R-wave progression.

Evidence of Ischemia or Infarction

Anterior leads: There are no changes specific for ischemia or infarction.
Inferior leads: There are no changes specific for ischemia or infarction.

Summary

Normal sinus rhythm at 90 bpm
Intervals: 0.16/0.08/0.40
QRS axis: +15 degrees
Left atrial enlargement

CASE 58 □ 179

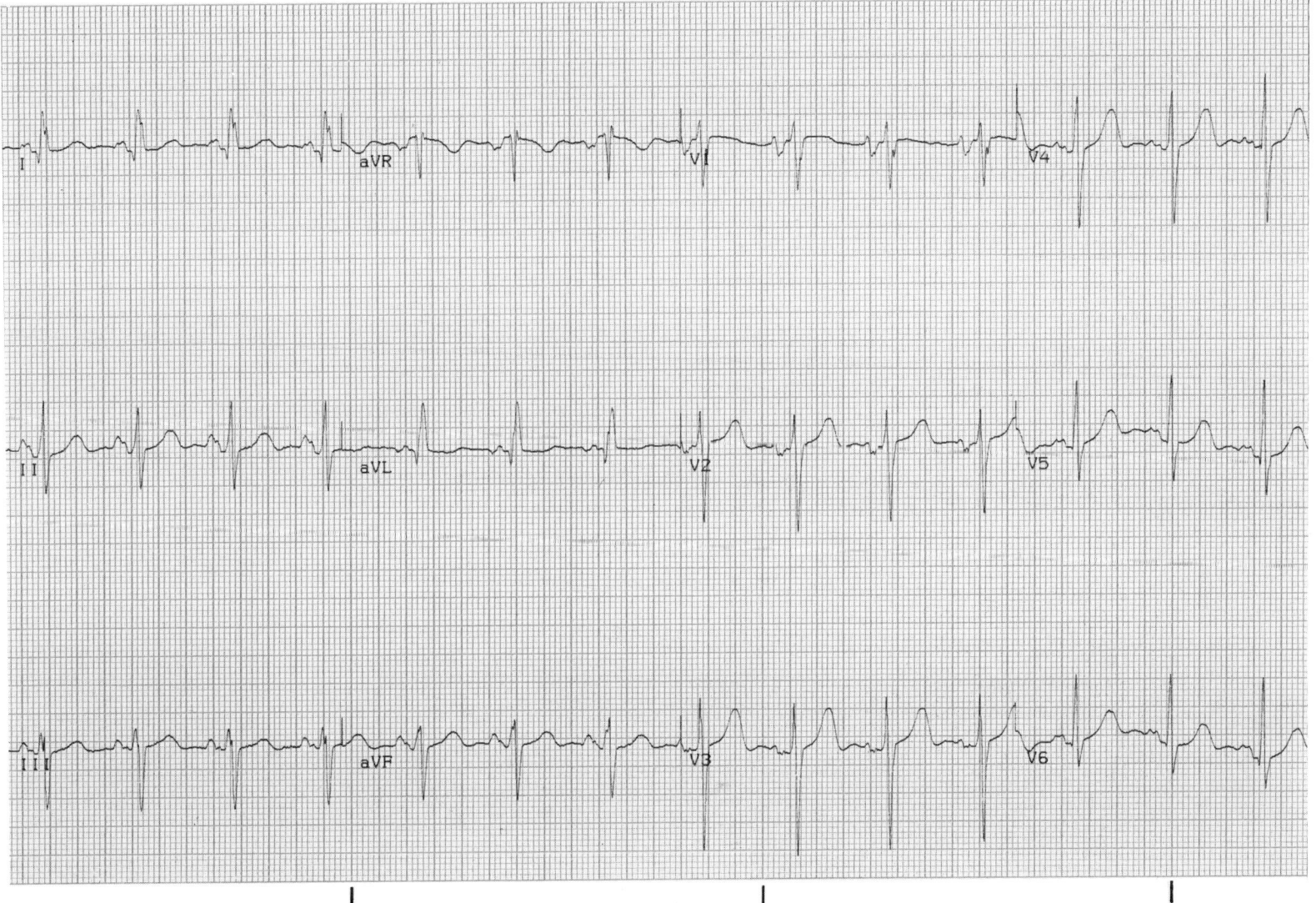

CASE 59

Rate and Rhythm

There is a P wave preceding each QRS complex, and the rhythm is normal sinus rhythm.

The heart rate is about 85 beats per minute.

Intervals

PR interval: 0.16s
QRS duration: 0.12s
QT interval: 0.36s

The prolonged QRS duration indicates that there is a bundle-branch block. Examination of V1 shows a QRS complex typical of left bundle-branch block.

QRS Axis

The QRS complex is positive in lead I and positive in lead aVF, so the QRS axis is in the normal quadrant. Leads III and aVF are closest to isoelectric, so the QRS axis is between +30 and 0 degrees, or about +15 degrees.

Evidence for Atrial Enlargement

In lead II, the P waves are notched and widened to more than 2.5 mm. In lead V1, the P waves are biphasic, with the terminal part wider than 1 mm. Thus there is left atrial enlargement.

Evidence for Ventricular Hypertrophy

In the presence of left bundle-branch block, we cannot assess for evidence of ventricular hypertrophy.

R-Wave Progression

In the presence of left bundle-branch block, we cannot assess R-wave progression.

Evidence of Ischemia or Infarction

In the presence of left bundle-branch block, we cannot assess for evidence of ischemia or infarction.

Summary

Normal sinus rhythm at 85 bpm
Intervals: 0.16/0.12/0.36
QRS axis: +15 degrees
Left atrial enlargement
Left bundle-branch block

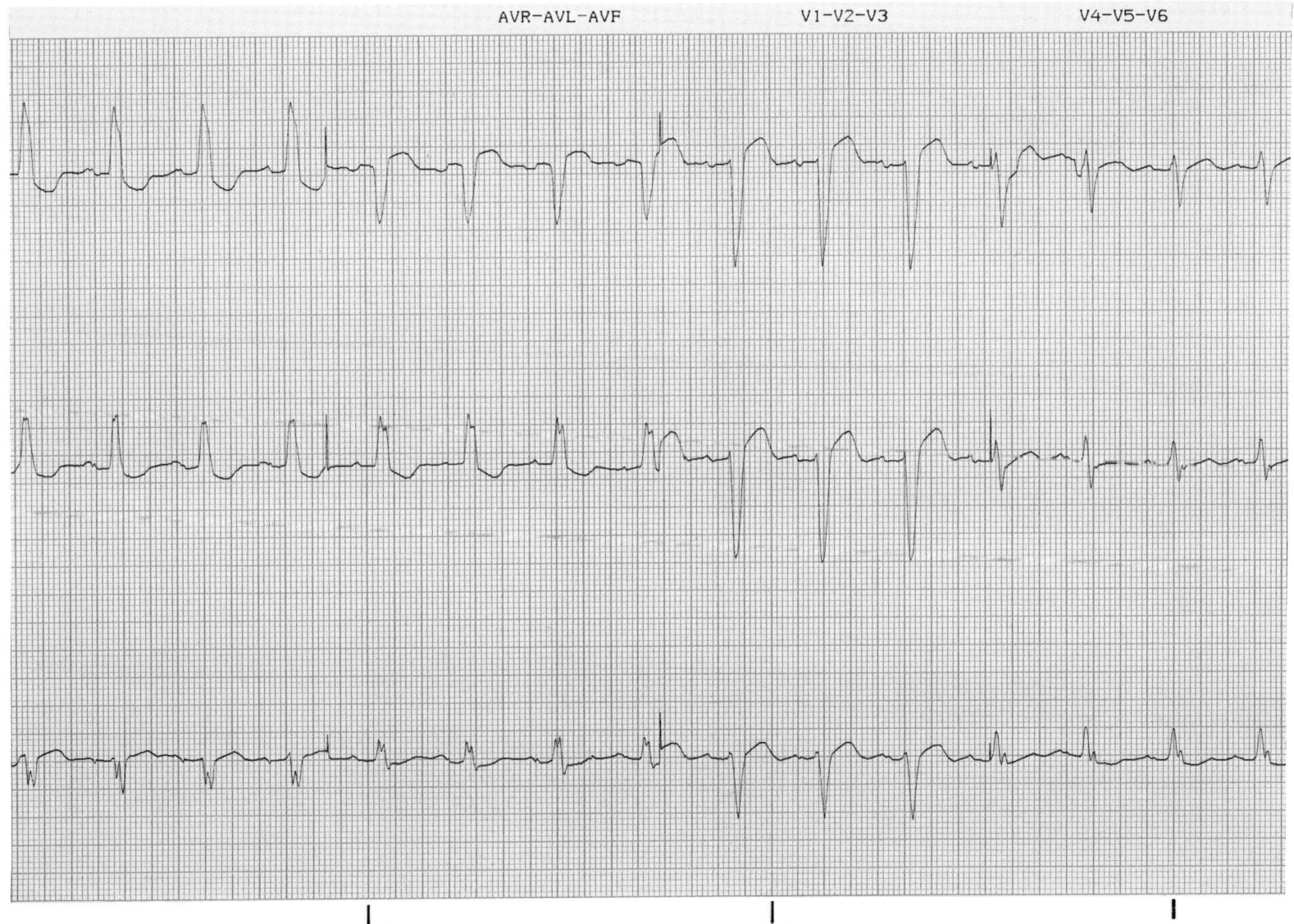

CASE 60

Rate and Rhythm

There is a P wave preceding each QRS complex, and the rhythm is normal sinus rhythm.

The heart rate is 95 beats per minute.

Intervals

PR interval: 0.16s
QRS duration: 0.06s
QT interval: 0.32s

QRS Axis

The QRS complex is positive in lead I and positive in lead aVF, so the QRS axis is in the normal quadrant. Leads III and aVF are closest to isoelectric, so the QRS axis is between +30 and 0 degrees, or about +15 degrees.

Evidence for Atrial Enlargement

The P waves are notched in lead II, but they are not widened to 2.5 mm. This tracing does not meet criteria for atrial enlargement.

Evidence for Ventricular Hypertrophy

LVH: The sum of the S wave in V1 (8 mm) and the R wave in V5 (7 mm) is 15 mm. There is no evidence of left ventricular hypertrophy by voltage criteria. The QRS voltage is low, being less than 5 mm in most of the limb leads and less than 15 mm in the precordial leads.

RVH: The QRS axis is in the normal quadrant. There is no evidence for right ventricular hypertrophy.

R-Wave Progression

The R waves do not grow very much from V1 to V4. There is poor R-wave progression.

Evidence of Ischemia or Infarction

Anterior leads: There is poor R-wave progression. The T waves are biphasic to inverted in V2 to V6 and I. This is consistent with anterior ischemia or subendocardial infarction.

Inferior leads: There are nonspecific ST-T wave abnormalities.

Summary

Normal sinus rhythm at 95 bpm
Intervals: 0.16/0.06/0.32
QRS axis: +15 degrees
Low voltage consistent with pericardial effusion, hypothyroidism, or chest wall abnormality
Poor R-wave progression with biphasic to inverted T waves in leads V2 to V6 and I consistent with anterior ischemia or infarction
Nonspecific ST-T wave abnormalities

CASE 60 □ 183

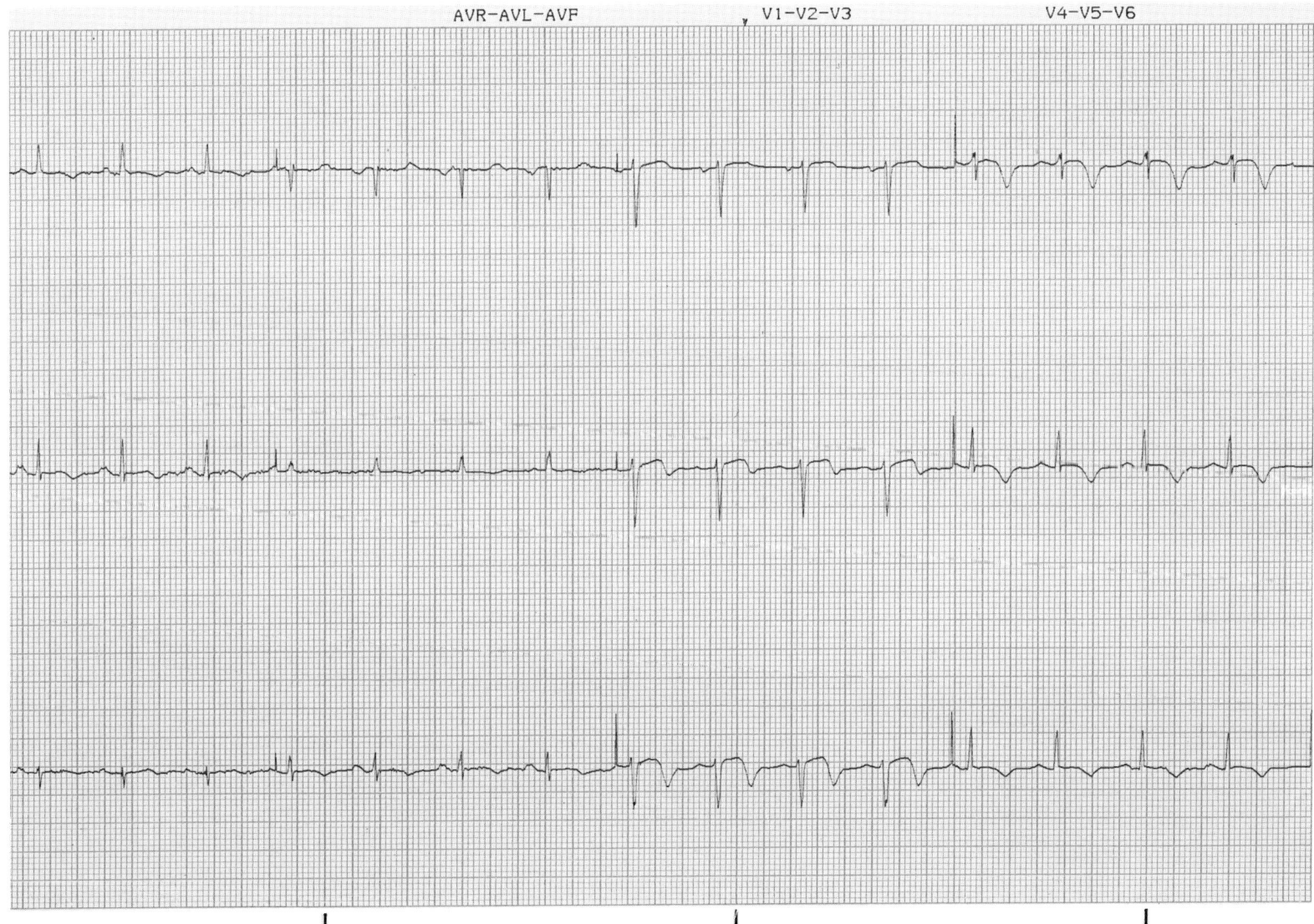

INDEX

Note: Page numbers in *italic* refer to illustrations.

Aberrancy, 55–56
Accelerated idioventricular rhythm (AIVR), 55
Antidepressants, 58
Arrhythmias, approach to, 37–38
    supraventricular, 43–51
    ventricular, 53–55
Artery(ies), coronary, anatomy of, 29–30
Ashman beats, 56
Atrial enlargement, 15–18
Atrial fibrillation (AF), 49
Atrial flutter, 48
Atrial pacemaker, low, 45
    wandering, 46
Atrial premature beats, 44, *45*
Atrial rhythms, 43–49
Atrial tachycardia, multifocal, 46
    paroxysmal, 47
Atrioventricular (AV) blocks, 38–40
Atrioventricular (AV) dissociation, 40
Atrioventricular (AV) node, in heart activation, 21
Atrium, activity of, in approach to arrhythmias, 37–38
    enlargement of, signs of, in reading ECGs, 36
Automaticity, in approach to arrhythmias, 38
AVL voltage criterion, for left ventricular hypertrophy, 19
Axis, 36
    horizontal, time measured on, 5
    QRS, 9–11
    vertical, voltage measured on, 5

Beats, Ashman, 56
    escape, 38
    premature, 38
        atrial, 44, *45*
        ventricular, 53
Bigeminy, 54
Blood supply, to heart, anatomic distribution of, 29–30
Bradycardia, sinus, 43, *44*

Bundle-branch block(s), 22
    left, 24
    patterns of, 22–26
    right, 25

Complexes, 7
    premature ventricular, 53–54
    QRS. See *QRS complex*.
Coronary arteries, anatomy of, 29–30

Digitalis, 57–58
Drugs, 57–58

Effusion, pericardial, 61
Electrical alternans, in pericardial effusion, 61
Electrodes, 4–5
Electrolyte abnormalities, 59–60
    T-wave inversions in, 32
Escape beats, 38
Estes scoring system, for left ventricular hypertrophy, 19, *20*

Fibrillation, atrial, 49
    ventricular, 54

Gallbladder disease, T-wave inversions in, 32

Heart, activation of, normal, 21–22
    blood supply to, anatomic distribution of, 29–30
    rotation of, R-wave progression and, 12–13
Heart block, complete, 40
    first-degree, 39
    second-degree, 39
    third-degree, 40
Heart rate determination, 5–6

Hemiblocks, *26*, 27
His-Purkinje system, 22
Horizontal axis, time measured on, 5
Hypercalcemia, 60
Hyperkalemia, 59
Hypertrophy, ventricular, 19–20
Hypocalcemia, 60
Hypokalemia, 59

Idioventricular rhythm, 55
Infarction, 31–33. See also *Myocardial infarction*.
Intervals, 7–8
Ischemia, patterns of, 31–33

Junctional escape, 50
Junctional rhythms, 50
Junctional tachycardia, 50

Leads, anatomic groups of, 30, *31*
    chest, appearance of QRS complex in, 12
    standard, 3
Left anterior hemiblock (LAHB), *26*, 27
Left atrial enlargement (LAE), 15–16, 17–18
Left axis deviation (LAD), 11
Left bundle-branch block (LBBB), 24
Left main (LM) artery, 30
Left posterior hemiblock (LPHB), *26*, 27
Left ventricular hypertrophy (LVH), 19–20

Metabolic abnormalities, T-wave inversions in, 32
Multifocal atrial tachycardia (MAT), 46
Myocardial infarction, evolution of, 33
    patterns of, 31–33
    posterior, reciprocal changes in, 32–33
    Q-wave, 33
    subendocardial, 32, 33
    transmural, 33

Myocardial ischemia, patterns of, 31–33
  signs of, in reading ECGs, 36

Neurologic damage, T-wave inversions in, 32
Non-Q-wave infarction, 32, 33

P waves, 7
  in lead II, in atrial enlargement, 16–17
  in lead VI, in atrial enlargement, 17–18
Pacemaker, atrial, low, 45
  wandering, 46
Pacemaker centers, automaticity of, 38
Paroxysmal atrial tachycardia (PAT), 47
Paroxysmal supraventricular tachycardia (PSVT), 47
Pericardial effusion, 61
Pericardial processes, 60–61
Pericarditis, 60–61
Phenothiazines, 58
Polymorphous ventricular tachycardia, 55
Posterior myocardial infarction, reciprocal changes in, 32–33
PR interval, 8
Premature beats, 38
  atrial, 44, *45*
  ventricular, 53
Premature ventricular complexes (PVCs), 53–54

Q wave infarction, 33
Q waves, in myocardial infarction, 31
QRS axis, 9–11
QRS complex, 7
  appearance of, in chest leads, 12
  duration of, in tricyclic antidepressant overdose, 58
  in left bundle-branch block, 24
  in right bundle-branch block, 25

QRS complex *(Continued)*
  in ventricular arrhythmias, 53
  morphology of, in approach to arrhythmias, 38
  normal, 22, *23*
QRS duration, 8
QT interval, 8
Quinidine, 58

R wave progression, 12–13
R waves, loss of, in myocardial infarction, 31
Reciprocal changes, in myocardial infarction, 32–33
Rhythm(s), atrial, 43–49
  idioventricular, 55
  junctional, 50
  sinus, 43–44
Right atrial enlargement (RAE), 15–17, 18
Right axis deviation (RAD), 11
Right bundle-branch block (RBBB), 25
Right ventricular hypertrophy (RVH), 20
Rotation of heart, R-wave progression and, 12–13

Sinoatrial (SA) node, automaticity of, 38
  in heart activation, 21
Sinus bradycardia, 43, *44*
Sinus node, automaticity of, 38
Sinus rhythm, 43–44
Sinus tachycardia, 43, *44*
Sokolow and Lyon's voltage criterion, for left ventricular hypertrophy, 19
Strain pattern, in ventricular hypertrophy, 20
ST-segment, depression of, in myocardial ischemia, 32
  types of, *32*
  elevation of, in myocardial infarction, 31–32
ST-T wave abnormalities, nonspecific, 33
  secondary, in bundle-branch block, 25
Subendocardial myocardial infarction (SEMI), 32, 33

Supraventricular arrhythmias, 43–51
Supraventricular tachycardia (SVT), aberrant, ventricular tachycardia versus, 56
  paroxysmal, 47
Systematic approach, to reading ECGs, 35–36

T waves, 7
  in bundle-branch block, 25
  inversion of, in myocardial ischemia, 32
  pseudonormalization of, in subendocardial myocardial infarction, 33
Tachycardia, atrial, multifocal, 46
  paroxysmal, 47
  junctional, 50
  sinus, 43, *44*
  paroxysmal, 47
Time, horizontal axis measuring, 5
Torsades de pointes, 55
Transmural infarction, 33
Tricyclic antidepressants, 58
Trigeminy, 54

Ventricular arrhythmias, 53–55
Ventricular ectopic activity (VEA), 53–54
Ventricular fibrillation, 54
Ventricular hypertrophy, 19–20
Ventricular premature beat (VPB), 53
Ventricular tachycardia (VT), 54
  polymorphous, 55
  versus aberrant supraventricular tachycardia, 56
Vertical axis, voltage measured on, 5
Voltage, vertical axis measuring, 5

Wandering atrial pacemaker, 46
Wenckebach block, 39